THE CALDESI LOW-CARB CHRISTMAS

Celebrate with 40 low-carb and gluten-free recipes

Text copyright 2020
© Katie Caldesi
Photographs copyright 2020 © Phoebe Pearson
Design and layout 2020 © Phoebe Pearson

Katie Caldesi is hereby identified as the author of this work in accordance with Section 77 of the Copyright, Designs and Patents Act 1988.

All right reserves. No part of the work may be reproduced or utilized in any form or by any means, electronic or mechanical, including photocopying, recording or by any information storage and retrieval system, without the prior written permission of the publisher.

Medical Disclaimer
The information in this e-book is only part of how any particular person may decide which diet or indeed lifestyle is best for them. If you are on prescribed medication or suffer from a significant medical condition, we strongly advise you to consult your own doctor before making changes. For example, improvements in lifestyle and weight loss may also significantly improve your blood pressure or diabetes control requiring a reduction in medication.

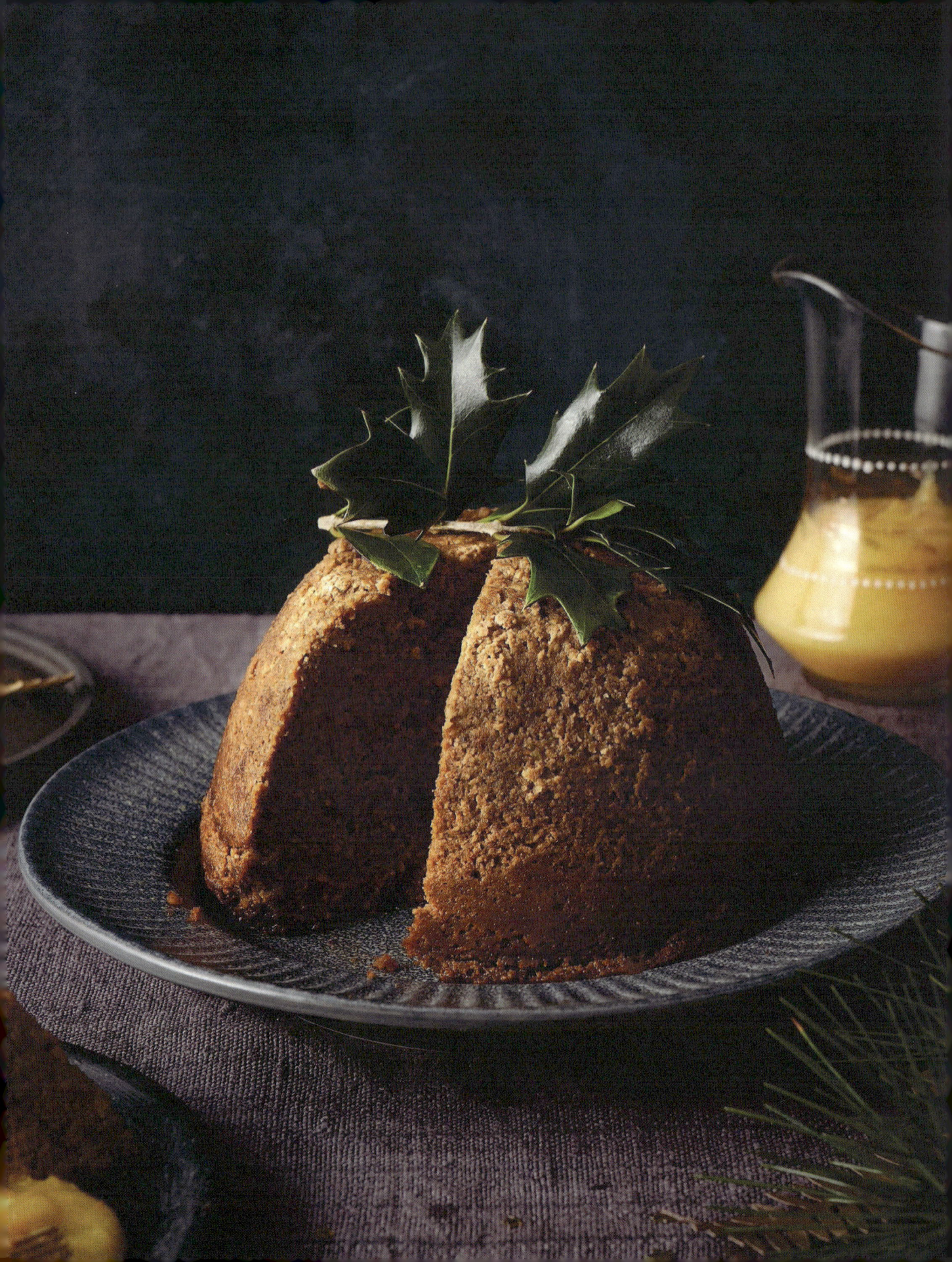

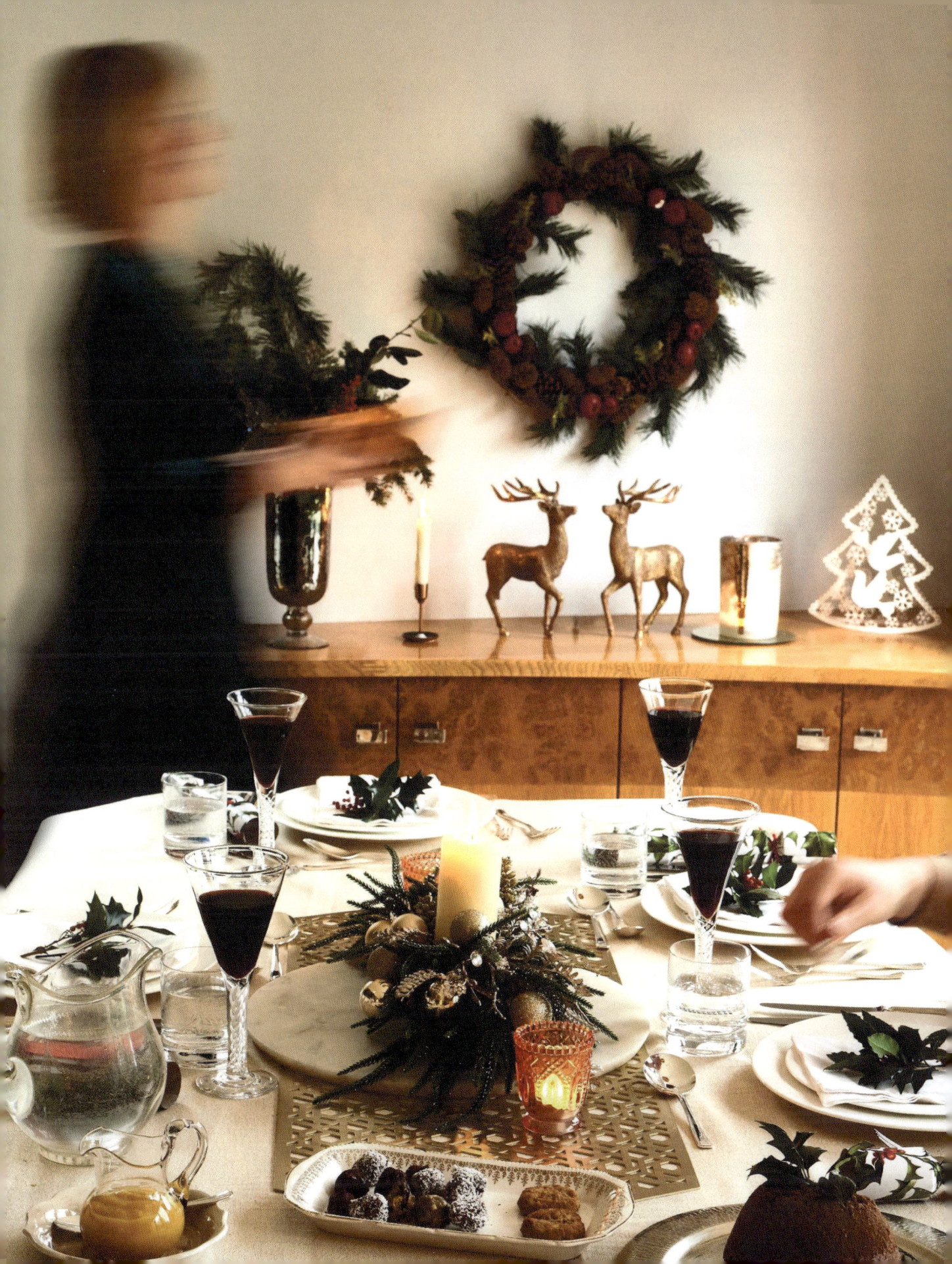

Contents

Foreword by Dr David Unwin — p7
Seven Top Tips for Christmas Cheer by Jenny Phillips — p8
Katie's Introduction — p10

CHAPTER 1 – STARTERS & CANAPÉS

1. Salmon, Avocado & Mango Ceviche — p17
2. Smoked Cheese & Cauliflower Soup — p19
3. Pizzette — p21
4. Crab, Tarragon & Avocado in Lettuce Shells — p23
5. Spinach, Smoked Salmon & Cream Cheese Spirals — p24
6. Oven-baked Ricotta with Rosemary & Shallots — p27

CHAPTER 2 – WINTERY LUNCHES & SUPPERS

7. Beetroot & Red Wine Risotto with Goat's Cheese Cream — p31
8. Chicken Thighs with Sage & Leek Cream Sauce — p33
9. Baked Fish with Red Pepper Sauce & Spicy Almonds on Roast Vegetables — p35
10. Malaysian Beef Rendang — p37
11. Homity Pie — p39
12. Savoy Pasta with Hot-smoked Salmon, Cream & Chilli Vodka — p41

SIDE DISHES

13. Sage & Onion Stuffing Cake — p45
14. Mashed Swede — p47
15. Celeriac & Swede Dauphinoise — p49
16. Stir-fried Sprouts with Onion, Bacon & Walnuts — p51
17. Roasties — p52
18. Cranberry Sauce — p53
19. "Bread" Sauce — p54
20. The Gravy — p55
21. Cauliflower Rice — p56

CHAPTER 3 – BREAD, PASTRY & CRACKERS

22. Multi-seed Crackers — p58
23. Caraway & Walnut Baguettes — p59
24. A Festive Ring of Rolls — p61
25. Sausage Rolls — p63

CHAPTER 4 – DESSERTS & SWEET TREATS

26. Pumpkin Porridge — p67
27. Coconut, Rum & Lime Trifle — p69
28. Vanilla Custard — p70
29. Christmas Cookies — p71
30. Chocolate Yule Log — p73
31. Spiced Christmas Pudding with Hot Marmalade Sauce — p76
32. Marmalade — p77
33. Mince Pies — p79
34. Chocolate Truffles — p81/82

CHAPTER 5 – COCKTAILS & DRINKS

35. Ginger Sparkler — p85
36. Lime Soda — p85
37. Glühwein — p86
38. Whisky Oddball — p86
39. Smoky Mary — p87
40. Wonky Madonna — p89
41. Eggnog — p91

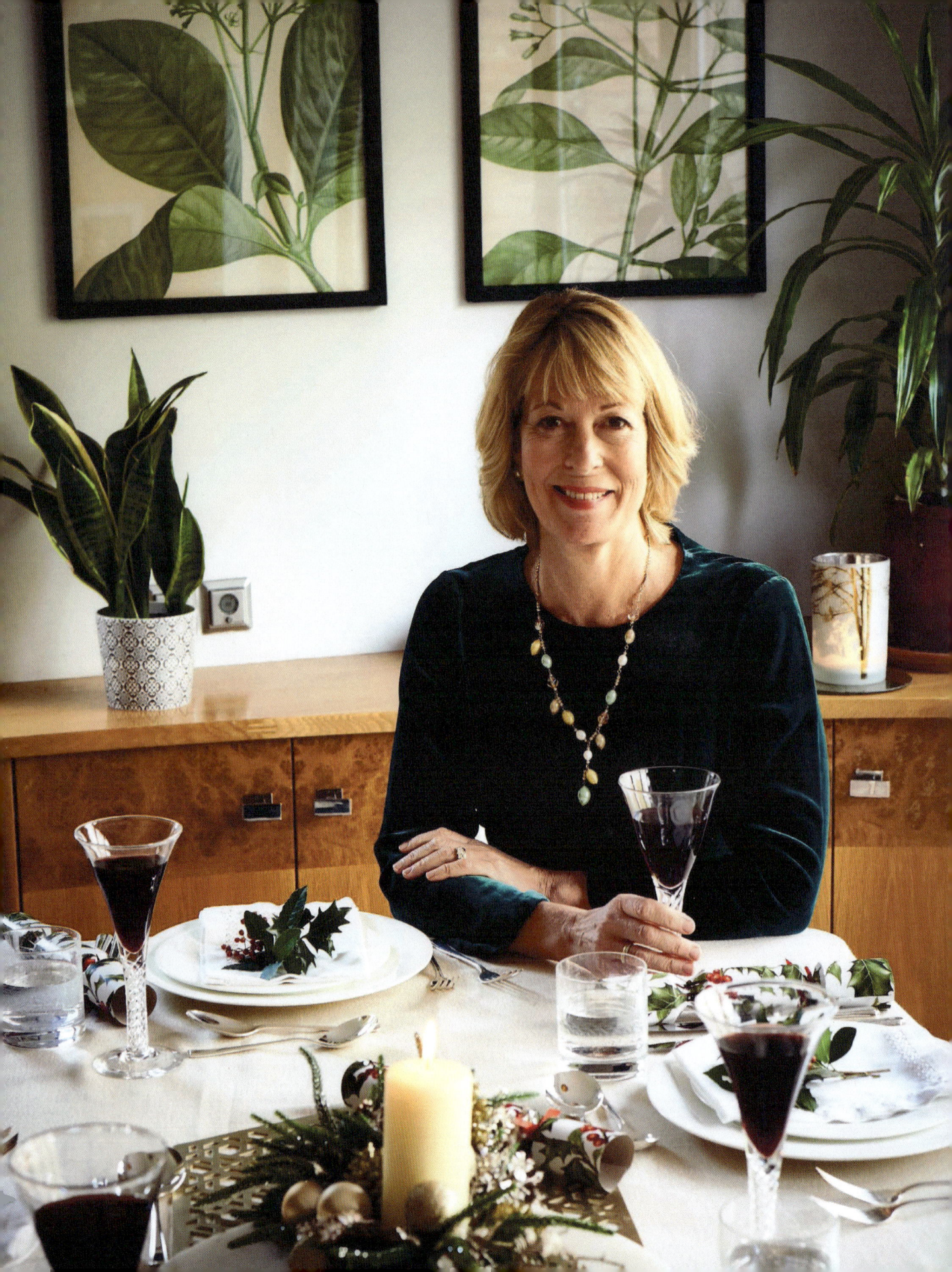

Foreword by Dr David Unwin FRCGP

GP and diabetes specialist, collaborator on our low-carb books Dr David Unwin explains how he prepares for Christmas.

Christmas, ah Christmas: mince pies, Christmas cake, boxes of chocolates, trifle. So many delicious food traditions built up from childhood. Does going low carb mean you will never enjoy Christmas ever again? Unthinkable!

"It's only one day". Be honest, is it? In my case until 2012, Christmas began with drinking sugary sloe gin in the weeks leading up to the big event. Usually, I had eaten all the chocolates off the tree in days and was forced to restock at least once. Meanwhile, in my GP practice patients' generosity meant tins of Quality Street and mince pies on tap in reception. Day by day I would notice my hunger ramp up, while at the same time I would become more tired in the evenings and need little naps, so that life was an effort. Then after Christmas it took me until March to get my weight and metabolism back to normal. Quite a sacrifice for just one day. It never occurred to me there was an alternative.

Even when I was first low carb, I felt I couldn't expect my family to sacrifice their Christmas to help me stay healthy. (Slightly odd sentiment now I think about it.) This resulted in a total derailing of my diet that took months to repair. I have noticed a very similar thing with so many of my patients facing January overweight and depressed.

So, we finally determined to learn from our mistakes and plan for a successful Christmas in advance. This involves enjoying indulgent, special foods we cannot normally afford. We look for flavour and quality in our ingredients. Buy wild smoked salmon instead of farmed, try lobster or pasture-raised, properly aged rib of beef. Indulge in expensive charcuterie, freshly cut instead of in plastic packs or unusual cheeses and walnuts in the shell. My wife Jen has learned to make pâté and low-carb trifle and I can bone and stuff a turkey with duck breasts, eggs and a meaty sage stuffing. Add in Bollinger Champagne or expensive red wine and malt whisky and Christmas begins to look a whole lot better!

So that's some low-carb Christmas ingredients sorted, now it's over to Katie Caldesi to give you the recipes. Merry (low-carb) Christmas!!

David

Dr David Unwin FRCGP @lowcarbGP

Seven Top Tips for Christmas Cheer by Jenny Phillips

Our www.lowcarbtogether.com nutritionist and co-author gives us her top tips.

Christmas is a time of fun and frivolity, with food and friends taking centre stage. It can be daunting to "diet" over this period and high expectations can result in feelings of disappointment (which often then perpetuates comfort eating). Here are some tips to keep you maxing out on fun and not calories this festive season.

1. Stay in control – It takes just a few minutes in the morning to consider the day ahead and make decisions about how you are going to play the day. What's going on? Where do you have to be? Who will be there? What sort of foods/drinks will be there to tempt you? Decide up front how much leniency to have and stick to it. Call this your "allowance" – a pre-agreed maximum for yourself.

2. Beware of the carbs – Christmas dinner is a synch – you should be able to fill up on protein and vegetables with maybe the odd parsnip or roast potato as a treat! The bigger danger area is puddings, which is where Katie's recipes give you alternative low-carb options without sacrificing any of the pleasure.

3. Alcohol – It has such a pull for many of us and, once it's reeled us in, it can be tough not to go overboard. So be aware and stick to the "allowance" you've agreed with yourself. Some useful tips for you: alternate drinks with glasses of water, offer to drive (and not drink), ask for spritzer (add fizzy water to white wine) and generally just pace yourself and keep hydrated.

4. Alcohol is probably the only beverage not to carry a nutritional label so you can be quite unaware that wine can clock up 185 calories per glass (250ml/9fl oz) and one pint of lager up to 247 calories. Be especially careful with liqueurs, which can deliver a massive injection of sugar. Instead, check out the cocktails and drinks chapter for low-carb friendly options.

5. Journaling – If the going gets tough and you feel that you have eaten too many carbs, keep a journal. Think of it as training your subconscious brain. Reflect on things you have done well, how you feel and what you've achieved. Record when things go off track – were there any triggers? What did you do? What different choices could you make next time? In this way you are reinforcing the behaviour you want and learning strategies for the future.

6. Missing meals – If you're not hungry, or you get up way too late for breakfast, then brunch can suffice. Feeling full from a big lunch? Then it's fine to skip the evening meal or have just a light bite. Intermittent fasting is a really effective way to reduce your calorie intake, without compromising on the quality of your food.

7. Clear your head – If you're feeling a little stodgy, get out for a brisk walk or some other exercise. Enjoy! Food is a pleasure and whichever choices you make, savour them.

Jenny

Jenny Phillips
Nutritional Therapist www.InspiredNutrition.co.uk

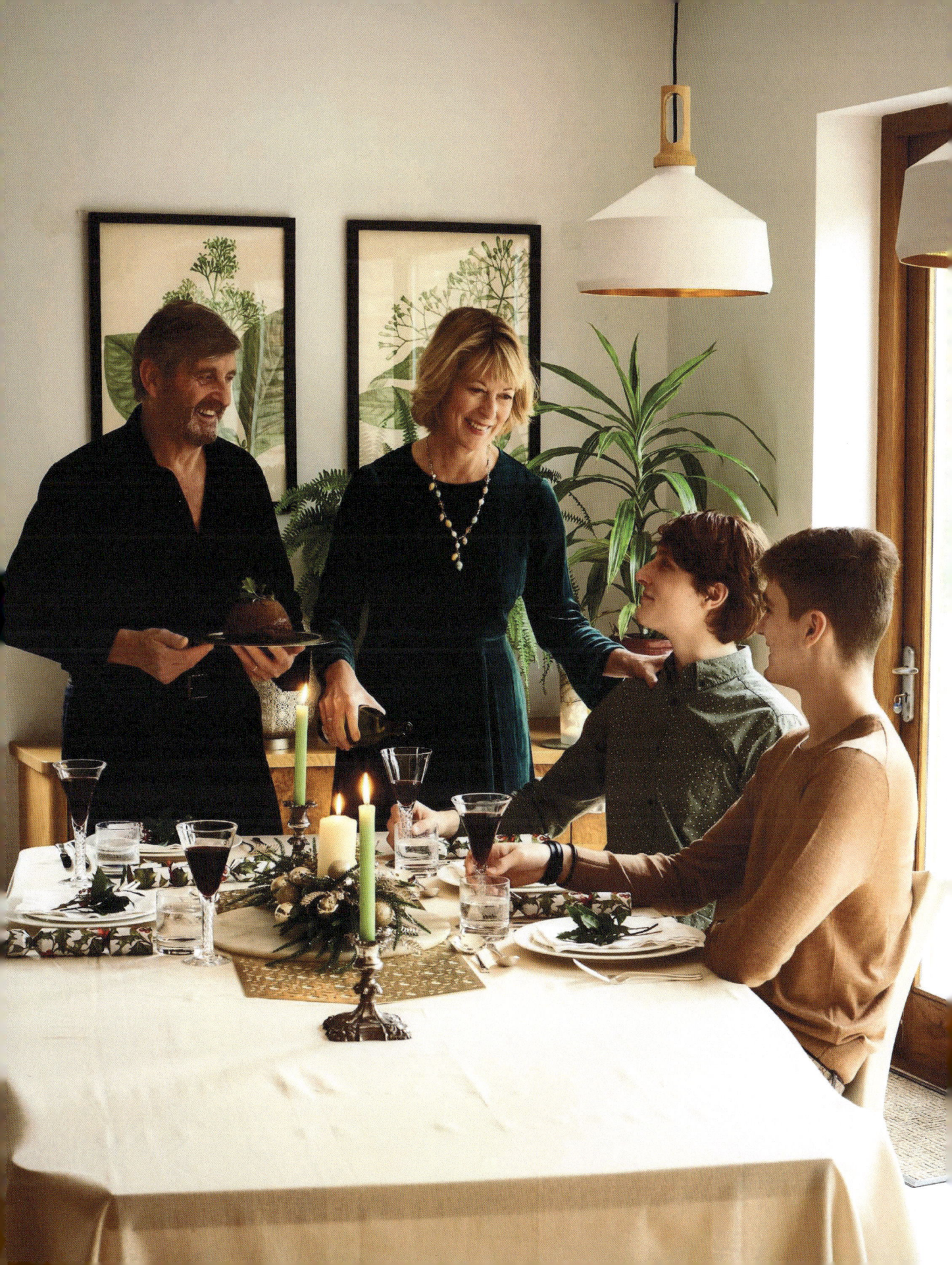

Katie's Introduction

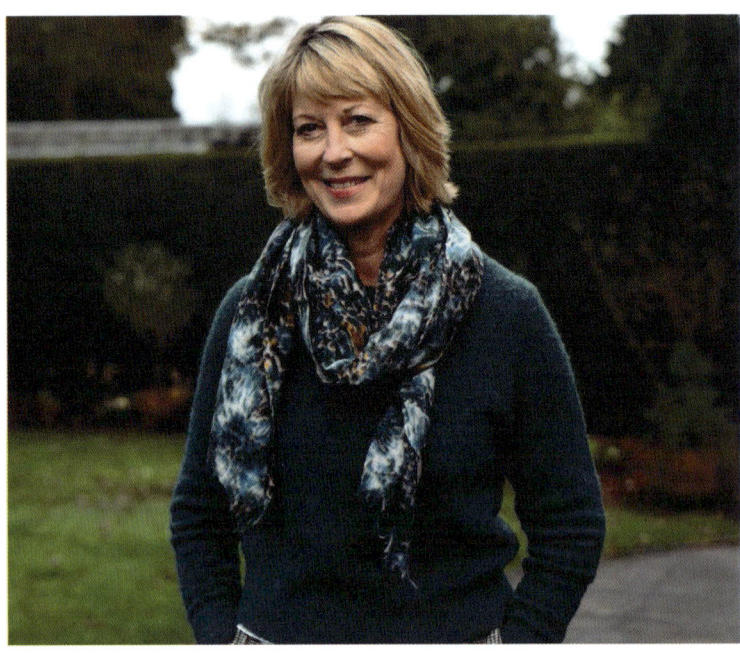

At the time of writing, we are in a second national lockdown so can't know quite how we will be celebrating Christmas and New Year this particular year. We don't know if our Italian restaurants will be open for business, whether we will be running them as takeaways or if we will be teaching cooking from our schools or over Zoom. However, we do know that we and our customers will want to celebrate. We will want to prepare traditional festive foods, enjoy comfort food to warm our bodies and souls after wintery walks and perhaps try out new recipes as treats over the holiday period. But we also know that we don't want to pile on the pounds.

At special times of the year, we give ourselves permission to overindulge, in fact it is positively expected of us. We like to feel "stuffed as a turkey" as the saying goes. All of this is fine once in a while if we are fit, lean and active but many of us aren't – in the UK 60% of us are obese and 1 in 15 people over 50 have type 2 diabetes. Overindulgence is the last thing we need.

My Italian chef husband, Giancarlo, is in remission from type 2 diabetes. Over the last 8 years we have followed a low-carbohydrate lifestyle for weight-loss and improved glucose control. He has brought his HbA1c (blood sugar levels) down from 79 mmol/mol to 39 mmol/mol so he is well within the normal range. Giancarlo has lost nearly 4 stone and I dropped the stone that always worried me. You can read his story and the science behind the low-carb lifestyle on our website www.lowcarbtogether.com.

We don't call going low-carb a "diet" as if it is something temporary. We are in it for life and love feeling this way; we are full of energy, lean and active. Our light-bulb moment was realizing that starchy foods break down into sugar in the body. Giancarlo knew he had to avoid sugar as a diabetic, but it wasn't until he restricted starchy foods that he made such amazing progress. We say he is "carb intolerant". Giancarlo can never go back to eating large amounts of pasta, potatoes, pastries, sugar, rice or sweets or he will become diabetic again. He was also diagnosed as gluten-intolerant, so all our low-carb recipes are gluten free too.

We have two sons and as a family we love food, cooking for friends, eating at our restaurants and going out to others. None of us would ever have been happy with low-calorie diet food, so it became my job to invent low-carb recipes that the whole family enjoyed. The low-carb lifestyle suits us all; we are not governed by gnawing hunger, we love the food that we eat and feel satiated but not stuffed. I strongly believe this book is for everyone as none of us need large amounts of sugar and refined carbs in our diet, ever. To decide for yourself how many carbs a day to eat, look at our quiz and [CarbScale](#) on our [site.](#)

I have written 15 cookbooks over the years but recently I have specialized in writing low-carb cookbooks – [The Diabetes Weight-loss Cookbook](#) and [The Reverse Your Diabetes Cookbook.](#) Our third book, [The 30 Minute Diabetes Cookbook,](#) is out in March 2021 and I am now writing a fourth book on the subject, so you could say I have become a low-carb expert.

In this ebook we show you how to avoid the usual carbs during Christmas. I have written recipes to help you with the festive canapés, starters, sides, bread, some main courses, drinks and even desserts and there are plenty more low-carb recipes on our website. I haven't included how to cook a turkey or the equivalent as the mains aren't usually the problem when avoiding carbs.

Sugar is so often bound up with traditional gifts throughout the year; it has become a way of showing our love for one another. In reality, if I give my husband a box of shop-bought chocolates as a gift it is a gentle way to give him a box of assorted poisons! It will shoot his blood sugar levels sky high and help him to gain pounds. Not such a nice present. As Dr David Unwin said earlier, we have found different ways of spoiling ourselves at Christmas rather than with sugar. This year we have a bottle of truffle oil which you will see I use to add a touch of winter luxury to foods. We have home-smoked a side of salmon to enjoy and we will be making the [chocolate truffles](#) to have on the Christmas table

Low-carb, gluten-free, keto and paleo

Our recipes are all low-carb and therefore suitable for the keto diet where net carbs are usually kept below 30g net carbs per day. If you are following a paleo diet where grains are avoided, and you eat some dairy, our gluten-free and grain-free recipes are good for you too.

A spoonful of sugar....

It is tricky with sweeteners as everyone has their own agenda and opinion and rightfully so. I see it as my job to give you options so you can make your own choices based on the following:

-are you cutting back on sugar as you believe that is how everyone should live?

-are you trying to lose weight quickly or you have gone keto?

-do you prefer to use artificial sweeteners?

-do you prefer to stay natural with honey, treacle or the natural sweetness of fruit?

We have used minimal honey or black treacle in the recipes but also given options for using erythritol, a sugar alcohol usually derived from corn, as I like the taste (I don't like the aftertaste of stevia). Erythritol has zero calories, doesn't impact your blood sugar levels and isn't harmful to dogs (xylitol is harmful to dogs).

We use both natural and artificial sweeteners in our household as although we want to cut right back on sugar, we do want flavour. I have had too many attempts at making recipes with no sugar only to have disappointed looks from my family as I serve them a cake that looks like a cake but doesn't taste like one. We have all adapted to low sugar but not no sugar. Experiment with how low you can go and do look at our website www.lowcarbtogether.com for more information on sweeteners.

Carb counts and nutritional analysis

Usually anyone following a low-carb diet will be looking for net carbs; that is total carbs minus fibre (which is insoluble). I use one to three forms of software to give me the nutritional analysis as they differ from one another at times. The values are only a guide and based on the ingredients I use. After a while, you "know" what is high carb and avoid those foods naturally, so you don't need to become obsessed with exact carb counts or calories.

Where I give a choice between using honey or treacle or erythritol, I have given the carb counts for two options - either using or excluding the honey or treacle. The latter assumes you will substitute your choice or sweetener (we prefer erythritol.) We don't show this in the nutritional analysis because it is misleading; sweeteners such as erythritol contain a type of carb called polyols or sugar alcohols which contain low or no calories, and don't affect blood sugar levels. Polyols are not absorbed by your body in the same way as sugar so although they look as high in carbs the effect on your body will be very different.

Suppliers

If you have difficulty sourcing ingredients or want to see which brands we prefer, take a look at our shop on our site www.lowcarbtogether.com

Most of all, enjoy the recipes and have fun cooking. We love to hear feedback as it helps us develop future recipes and ideas for our website; please contact me at info@lowcarbtogether.com.

We love to see your photos on social media too. Do tag me in so we can see and use #lowcarbchristmas if you like. We teach low carb cookery courses both on-line and in our schools in London, Gerrards Cross and Bray on Thames.

Happy Christmas

@katiecaldesi on Twitter
@katiecaldesi on instagram
@lowcarbtogether on Facebook

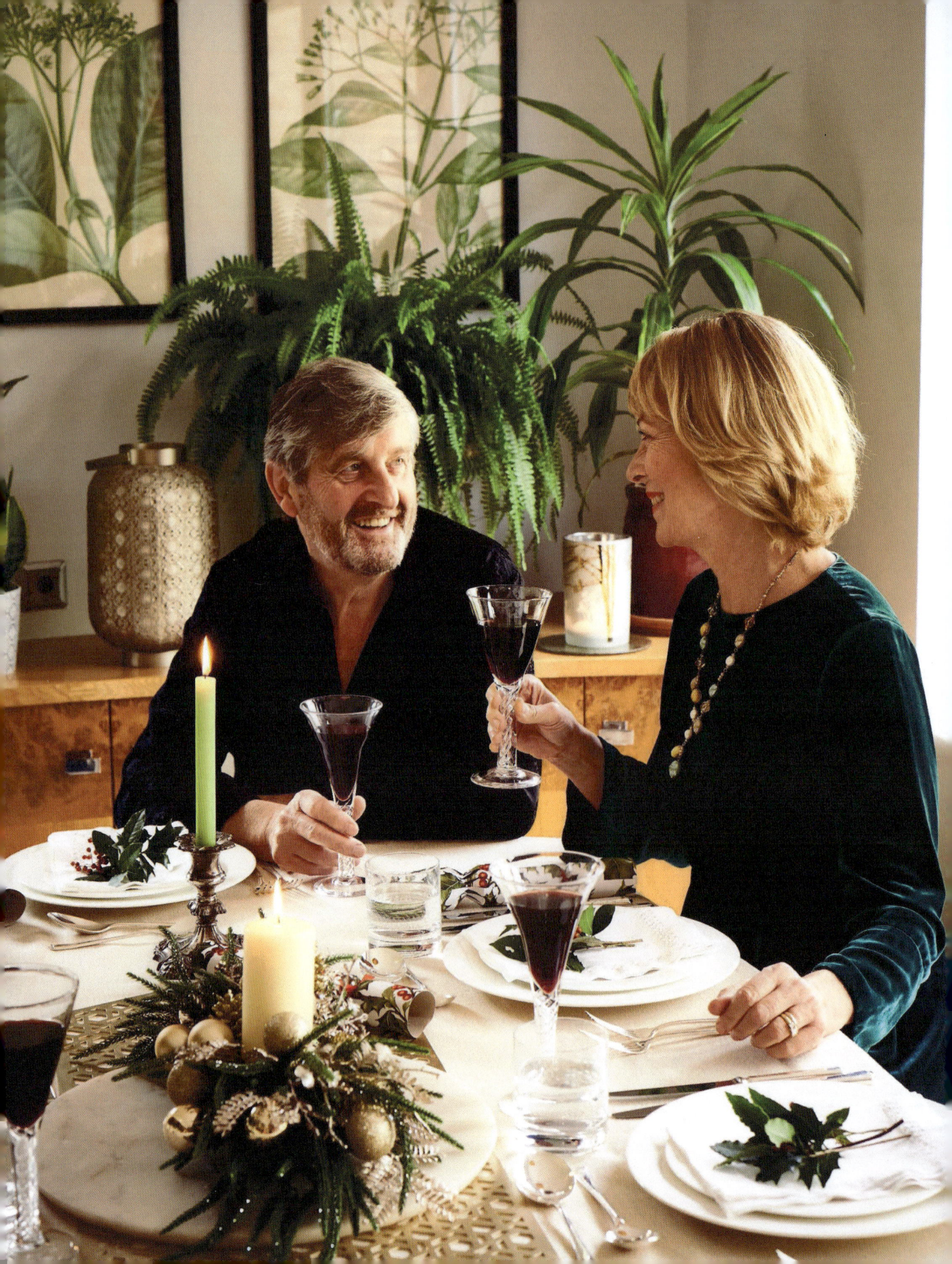

Chapter One

Starters & Canapes

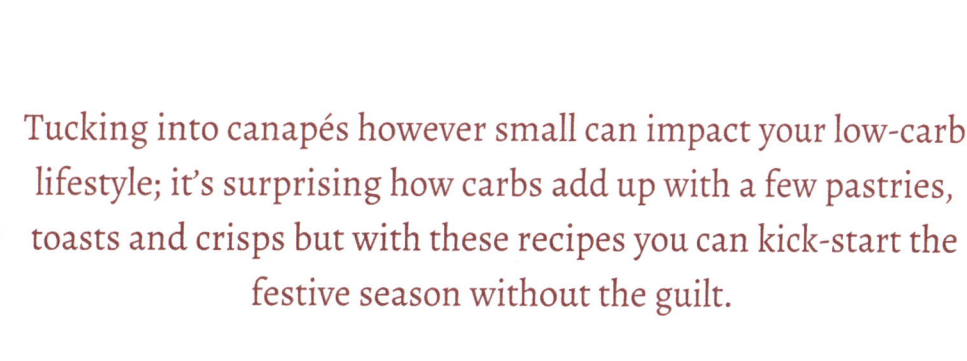

Tucking into canapés however small can impact your low-carb lifestyle; it's surprising how carbs add up with a few pastries, toasts and crisps but with these recipes you can kick-start the festive season without the guilt.

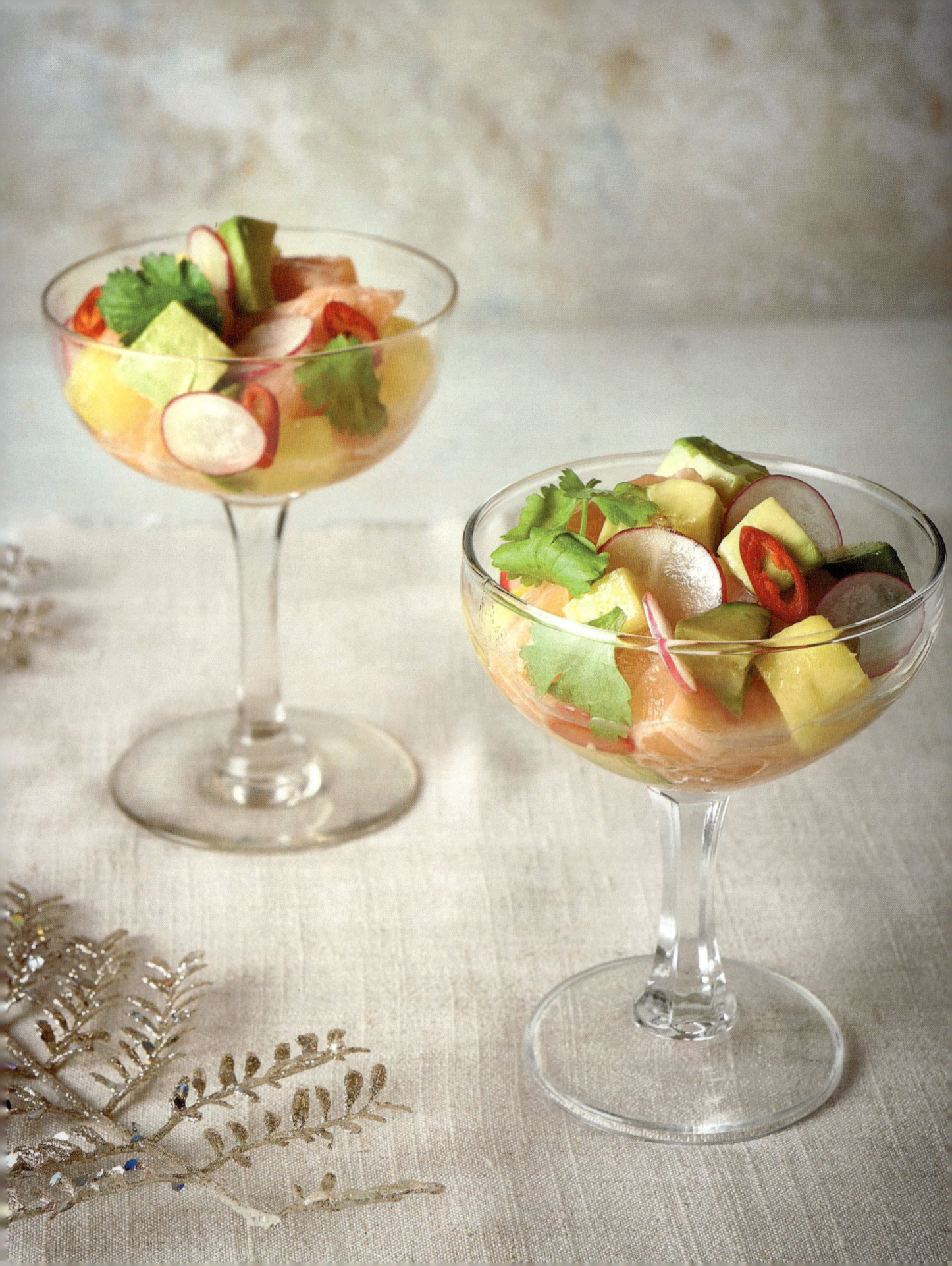

Salmon, Avocado & Mango Ceviche

This Peruvian classic can be a simple mixture of lime juice, chilli and salt poured over fish and fruit. It appears to "cook" the fish in minutes, turning it from translucent to opaque. What actually happens is that the proteins are denatured by the acid of the citrus fruit juice, giving the fish a cooked texture.

As the fish is not cooked with any heat, it is really important that the fish is "sushi-grade" fresh and safe to eat or that is has been commercially frozen at -20°C (-4°F) as this kills any possible parasites. This is difficult to do in a domestic freezer, but a good fishmonger can do this for you and a lot of fish sold in supermarkets has been previously frozen.

Fruit such as grapes, peach or mango are usually added to ceviche to give a welcome sweetness after the punchy citrus and salt. Lime is sometimes replaced with acidic passionfruit to do the same job. Tropical fruits are high in carbs and so we usually avoid them, but we have used a minimal quantity here; any remaining mango can be cut into cubes and frozen for use another day. Do taste your chilli so that you know how much to add. It is disappointing to not have enough of a kick of heat and overpowering to have too much! Any leftover radishes can go into the [Roasties.](#)

Serves 4

250g (9oz) fillets of salmon, tuna, swordfish or sea bass, pin-boned and skinned
150g (5½oz) mango flesh, cut into 1cm (½in) cubes
1 medium avocado, cut into 1cm (½in) cubes
2 radishes, finely sliced
¼–½ jalapeño chilli or hot green or red chilli, according to taste, finely sliced
1 teaspoon salt
a small handful of coriander leaves, roughly chopped
juice of 2 limes
2 spring onions, finely chopped

Soak the onions in cold water for 10 minutes to take the strength away, drain well. Gently mix the fish, fruit, vegetables and chilli together in a mixing bowl. Add the salt, coriander and lime juice and gently toss through. Divide between the serving dishes and serve straight away.

Per serving: 7.4g net carbs, 3g fibre, 13.9g protein, 8.1g fat, 164 kcal

Get ahead: Stop after mixing the fish, fruit and vegetables together and keep the bowl in the fridge, covered, for up to a day. Add the salt and lime just before serving.

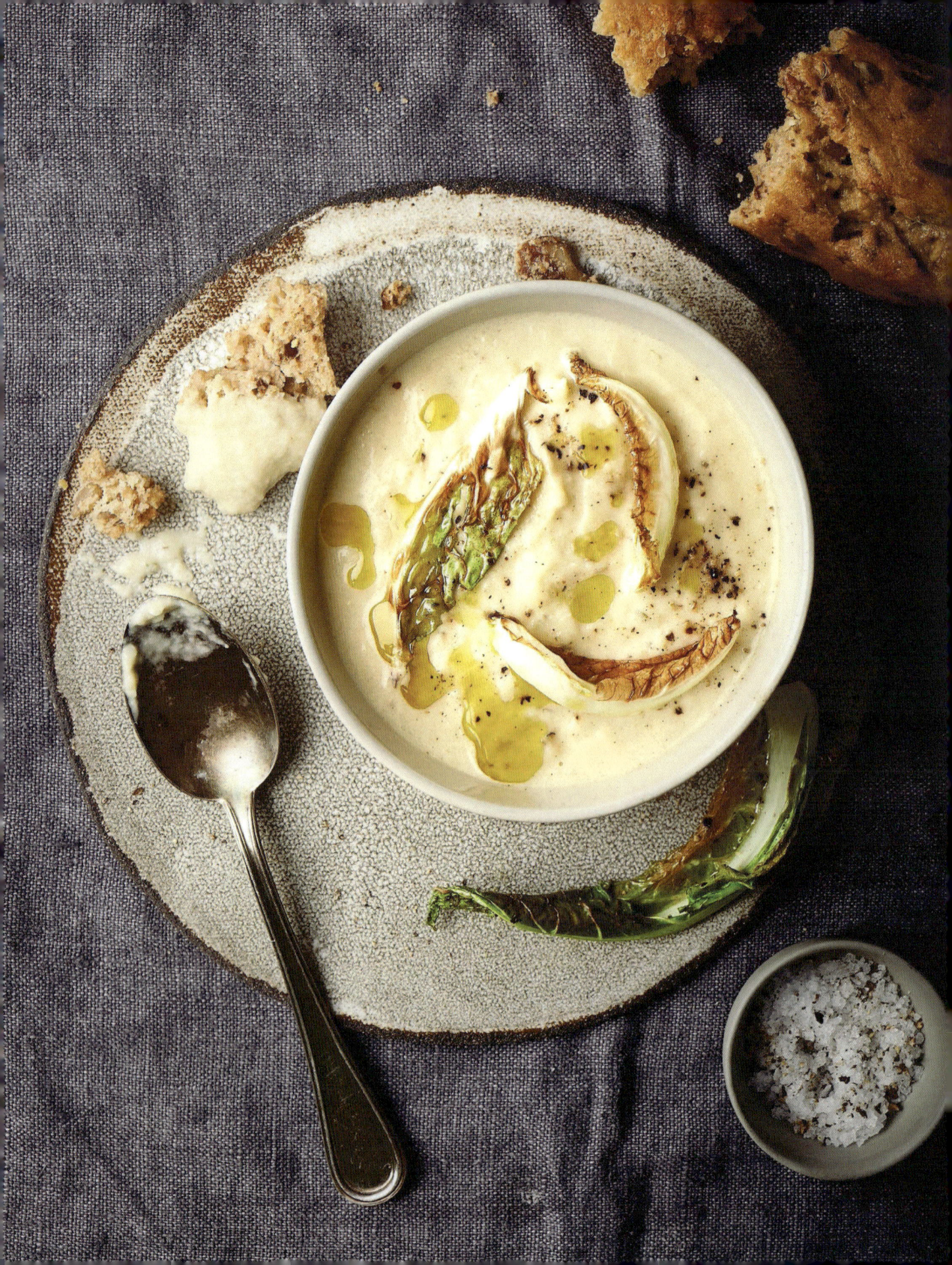

Smoked Cheese & Cauliflower Soup

This is a quick and simple soup that uses up ends of cheese left over in the fridge. We love the flavour of smoked Cheddar, but any cheese that melts will work, such as goat's or blue cheese. We like to add roasted cauliflower leaves on top. You can use broccoli instead of cauliflower. To be decadent at Christmas, try adding a swirl of truffle oil to the soup before serving.

Serves 6 as a starter and 4 as a main

3 tablespoons extra-virgin olive oil, ghee, butter or chicken fat
2 medium leeks (250g/9oz after trimming), roughly chopped
2 sprigs of thyme
600g (1lb 5oz) cauliflower, cut into small florets
1 litre (1¾ pints) warm vegetable stock, chicken stock or water
100ml (3½fl oz) double cream
125g (4 ¼ oz) smoked cheese, finely grated
2 tablespoons Dijon or 1 tablespoon English mustard
salt and freshly ground black pepper
extra virgin olive or truffle oil, to serve

Heat the oil in a large, heavy-based saucepan. Add the leeks and thyme and sauté for 10 minutes or until soft. Add the cauliflower, stock or water, mustard and bring to the boil. Continue to boil gently for a few minutes or until the cauliflower is tender. Remove the thyme sprigs and purée the soup with a stick blender or liquidizer until smooth, taking care the hot soup doesn't splash you.

Add the cream and cheese and stir over a low heat until the cheese has melted. Season to taste. Keep the soup warm while you prepare the cauli crisps.

When you are ready to serve, ladle the soup into warm bowls and scatter over the cauli crisps. Swirl over a little olive or truffle oil and add a twist of black pepper just before serving.

Cauli Crisps

Preheat the oven to 220° C/200 ° C fan/425° F/gas mark 7. Rub a little olive oil and seasoning into the cauliflower leaves and stems and spread them out on a baking tray. Roast for 4–6 minutes or until the leaves become lightly browned and crisp. Serve warm on their own or use to top the Smoked Cheese & Cauliflower Soup.

Per serving of soup as a main: 9.2g net carbs, 3.9g fibre, 12.4g protein, 35.2g fat, 406kcal
Per serving of soup as a starter: 6.1g net carbs, 2.6g fibre, 8.3g protein, 23.5g fat, 270kcal
Get ahead: The soup will keep in the fridge for up to 3 days, keep the leaves uncooked and pop them in the oven just before serving.

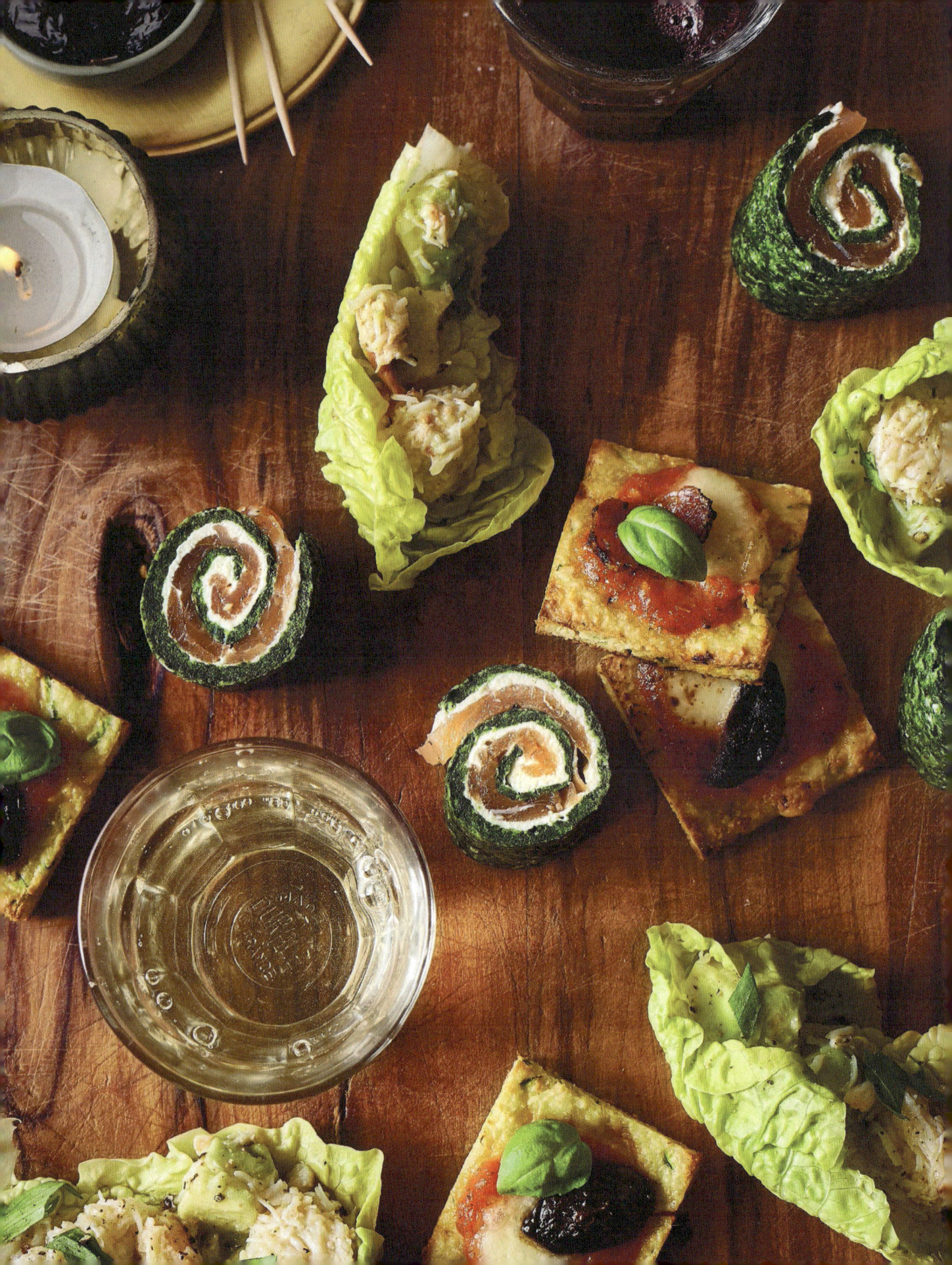

Pizzette

Our perfect pizza base is made from grated courgette and almonds. It forms a tasty and stable base for pizzas or pizzette – little pizzas. There is no rising time or tricky swirling of dough in the air, you simply stir, shape and cook! One top tip is to buy a basil plant for small leaves to decorate your pizzette. The basil sold in bags tends to have big leaves which will swamp small pizzette.

Makes approx. 32 pizzette or 2 pizzas

For the base
extra virgin olive oil, to grease
25g (1oz) Parmesan cheese
2 medium eggs
1 teaspoon salt
150g (5½oz) ground almonds
1 medium courgette (approx. 175–220g/6–8oz), peeled and coarsely grated

For the tomato sauce
100g (3½oz) passata or canned chopped tomatoes
1 teaspoon dried oregano
1 tablespoon extra-virgin olive oil
¼ teaspoon salt
freshly ground black pepper

For the topping
75g (2½oz) mozzarella, drained
A selection of the following:
a handful of olives, pitted
8–10 slices of salami
8 anchovies, drained of any oil
1 tablespoon extra-virgin olive oil, to finish
a few basil leaves, to finish

Preheat the oven to 200°C/180°C fan/400°F/gas mark 6. Line a large baking tray (about 30 x 30cm/12 x 12in or use two) with baking parchment and brush with oil.

Put all the ingredients for the pizza base in a bowl and mix together with a large metal spoon. It will form a fairly thick dough.

To make the pizzette, put the dough on to the prepared tray and use lightly oiled hands to press it out to a rectangle about 28 x 25 x 1cm (11 x 10 x ½in).

To make the pizzas, divide the dough in half and place on the prepared tray. Press and shape each piece with wet hands into a circle 1cm (½in) deep and 18–20cm (7–8in) in diameter. Bake for 10 minutes.

Meanwhile, blend the ingredients for the sauce together in a mixing bowl. Remove the tray from the oven and increase the temperature to 240°C/fan 220°C/475°F/gas mark 9 or as hot as it will go.

Cut the pizzette into 4cm (1½in) squares and gently move them apart from one another. If you aren't going to cook the pizzette or pizzas straight away, remove them from the baking tray to avoid them sweating underneath. They can be cooled and frozen at this point. When you are ready to cook the pizzette or pizzas, top each one with the tomato sauce, leaving a small border around the edge. Tear over the mozzarella and add the toppings of your choice.

Bake for 6–8 minutes until the mozzarella is bubbling and the crust is crisp and browned. Remove from the oven and serve straight away or allow to cool to room temperature. Scatter with the basil leaves just before serving.

Per pizzette with olive and salami: 0.5g net carbs, 0.6g fibre, 2.5g protein, 5g fat, 60kcal
Per pizza: 15.8g net carbs, 9.6g fibre, 39.4g protein, 80g fat, 969kcal

Get ahead: After the first 10 minutes of cooking, the bases can be cooled and kept in the fridge for 3 days or frozen for 3 months. Defrost before use.

Crab, Tarragon & Avocado in Lettuce Shells

This is the perfect light canapé to start off a party or an elegant starter to serve before a rich meal.

Serves 6/Makes 12 lettuce shells

3 Little Gem lettuces
100g (3½oz) white crabmeat
1 large avocado, sliced
a small handful of tarragon leaves, roughly chopped
2 tablespoons lemon juice
4 tablespoons extra virgin olive oil
salt and freshly ground black pepper

Cut the hard stem away from the lettuces. Carefully pull apart the leaves and choose the best of them for using as a container; use the rest in a salad another day. Lay the chosen ones on a serving dish or wooden chopping board.

Very gently toss the white crabmeat with the remaining ingredients. Season to taste. Spoon the crab into the lettuce cups, give them an extra twist of black pepper and serve straight away.

Per serving: 1.4g net carbs, 1.9g fibre, 2.9g protein, 12.6g fat, 132kcal

Get ahead: Make the crab mixture without adding the salt or herbs. It will keep for up to a day. Season to taste and add the tarragon just before filling the lettuce cups.

Spinach, Smoked Salmon & Cream Cheese Spirals

If you imagine a thin but strong spinach omelette, you will have got the gist of this versatile recipe. This was my answer to sheets of pasta when we became a gluten-free and low-carb household. I cut the spinach sheets into rectangles and used them in Giancarlo's beloved lasagne, cannelloni or a rotolo (a roulade-shaped baked pasta dish). Then a reader told me she used them as wraps– a great idea. Who needs the carbs from a flour wrap when you can have a spinach wrap instead?

We usually use bags of frozen spinach for this. They generally weigh 900g–1kg (2lb–2lb 4oz) and, to give you a guide, 900g (2lb) of frozen spinach becomes 300g (10½oz) once it is defrosted and squeezed well. Don't buy finely chopped spinach if you have the choice as it is harder to squeeze.

Makes 1 spinach sheet approx. 36 x 30cm (14¼ x 12in)/
Makes 16 spirals

extra virgin olive oil, to grease
approx. 150g (5½oz) defrosted spinach, squeezed dry from 450g (1lb) frozen spinach
½ teaspoon salt
2 medium eggs
4 tablespoons nut or cow's milk
2 teaspoons psyllium husk

For the filling
150g (5½oz) cream cheese
200g (7oz) smoked salmon
freshly ground black pepper

Preheat the oven to 220° C/200 ° C fan /425° F/gas mark 7, line a large baking tray with baking parchment and brush it with oil. Brush another sheet of baking parchment the same size with oil.

Blitz the spinach, salt, eggs, milk and psyllium husk powder together in a food processor to form a paste. Spoon the mixture on to the prepared tray. Put the piece of oiled baking parchment (oiled-side down) over the top and carefully press the spinach mixture out to form a thin rectangle measuring roughly 27 x 34cm (10¾ x 13¼in) and about 5mm (¼in) thick. Remove the top sheet of paper. (You can reuse it to wrap the spinach sheet if you don't use it straight away.) Tidy up the shape and even out the thickness using a flat-ended tool, such as a fish slice or dough scraper.

Bake for 8 minutes or until it is firm to the touch all over. Remove from the oven and leave to cool on the tray. The sheet can be rolled and covered with oiled baking parchment and either kept in the fridge for up to 3 days or frozen for 3 months.

To make the spirals, cut the spinach sheet into two long, slim rectangles about 15 x 28cm (6 x 11in). Leave them on the paper. Use a palette knife or spatula to spread the cream cheese evenly over the pieces leaving one long side with a border of 2mm (1/16in). Spread the salmon out over the top and add a twist of pepper. Use the paper to tightly roll the sheets into a spiral.

If time allows wrap the rolls in paper and transfer to the freezer for 30 mins to firm them up as they are easier to cut when cold. Use a serrated knife to cut them into 3cm (1¼in) lengths. Stand them up on a serving dish and serve straight away or cover and keep in the fridge for up to a day. Allow them 10 minutes to serve so that they are not fridge cold.

Per whole spinach sheet: 3.3g net carbs, 8.1g, 17.3g protein, 11.2g fat, 207kcal
Per spiral: 0.7g net carbs, 0.5g fibre, 3.9g protein, 4.5g fat, 60kcal

Get ahead: Make the sheets or the spirals in advance and chill or freeze them. Defrost before using.

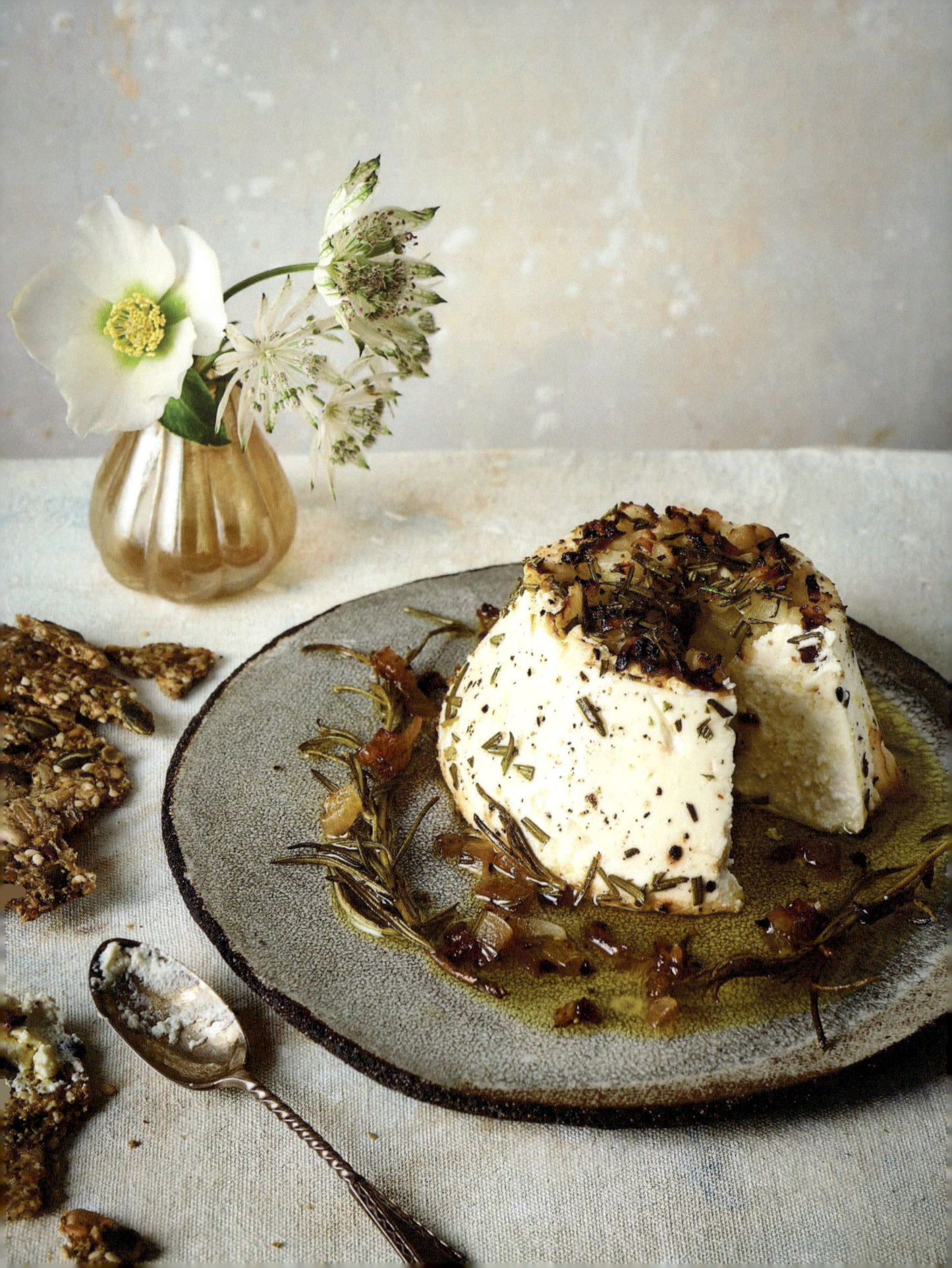

Oven-baked Ricotta with Rosemary & Shallots

We saw this dish at a Sicilian market in Palermo where a father and son were baking fresh ricotta in a tiny oven; the aroma of roasting onions and rosemary was enough to draw a crowd. It seemed such a simple idea and I couldn't wait to get home to try it. It's a brilliant recipe I keep returning to when I have people coming round. Buy the ricotta in one of those small plastic tubs to get the shape. If you can't find one like this, you can use a container and push the ricotta into it to work as a mould.

Change the herbs according to what you have – fresh or dried rosemary, thyme and sage transform the ricotta from bland to sublime. Serve the ricotta with low-carb bread, the [Multi-seed Crackers](#), sticks of vegetables or petals of chicory or baby lettuce.

Serves 6 as antipasti

250g (9oz) ricotta
3 sprigs of rosemary, needles removed from the stems and roughly chopped
1 shallot, finely chopped
3 tablespoons extra virgin olive oil
salt and freshly ground black pepper

Preheat the oven to 200°C/180°C fan/400°F/gas mark 6 and line a baking sheet with baking parchment.

Drain the ricotta and place on the prepared baking sheet. Gently push a dip into the top of the cheese, season, then scatter over the rosemary and chopped shallot, piling them up on top. Pour over the oil and bake for 20 minutes or until lightly browned. Serve while warm.

Per serving: 3.7g net carbs, 0.3g fibre, 3.4g protein, 11g fat, 126kcal

Get ahead: Prepare the ricotta with the flavourings and keep in the fridge; 20 minutes before your guests arrive pop it in the oven to bake. They will walk in to the aroma of a Sicilian market!

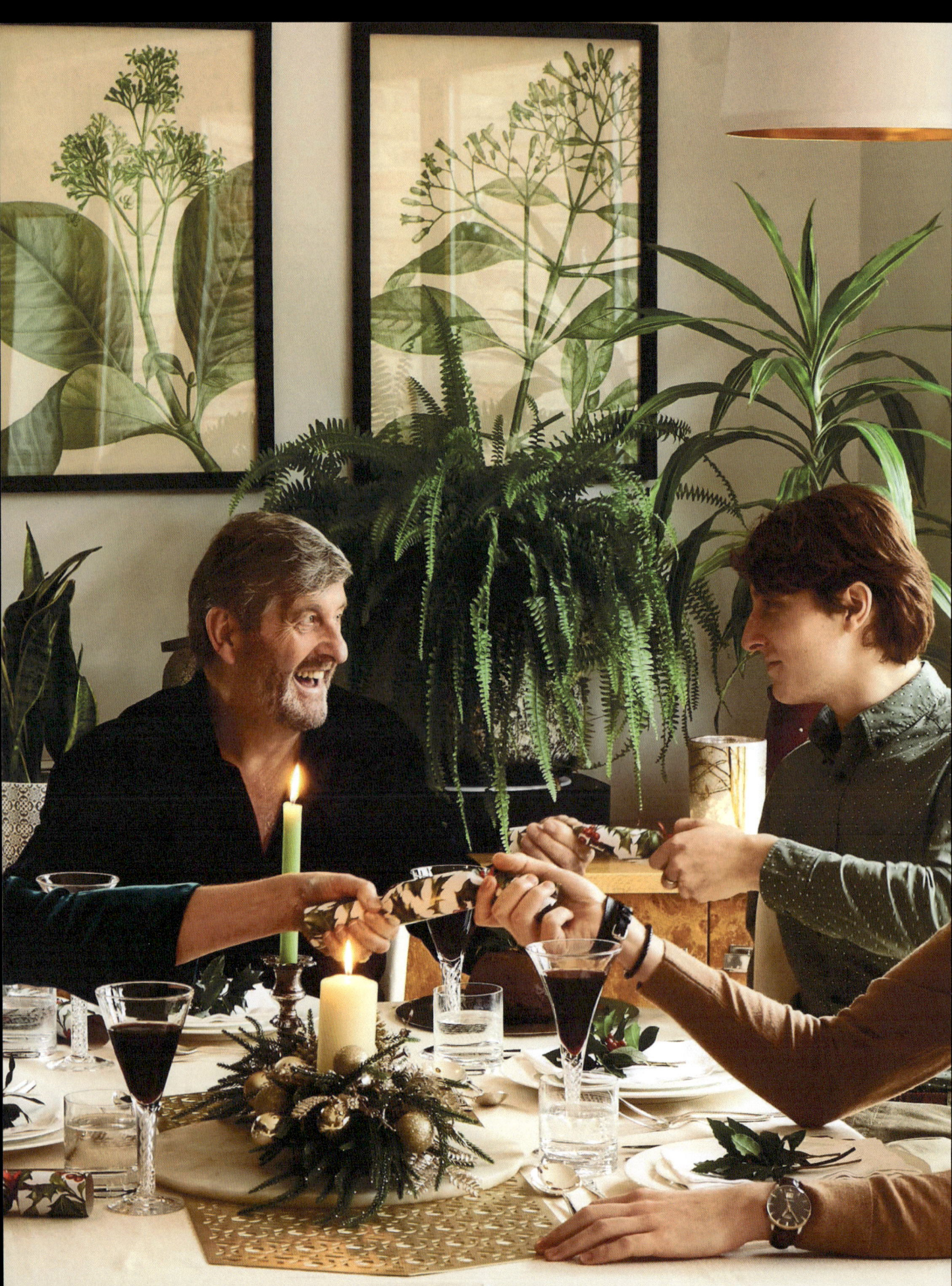

Chapter Two

Wintery Lunches & Suppers

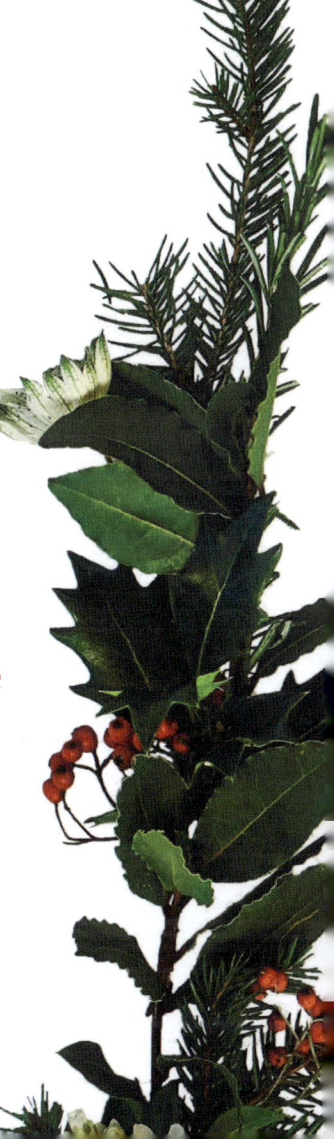

These main courses are full of flavour and will leave you satisfied but not sleepy. Each dish is made from or paired with a low-carb vegetable as an alternative to the usual Christmas carbs, so you won't miss the potatoes, rice and pasta, I promise!

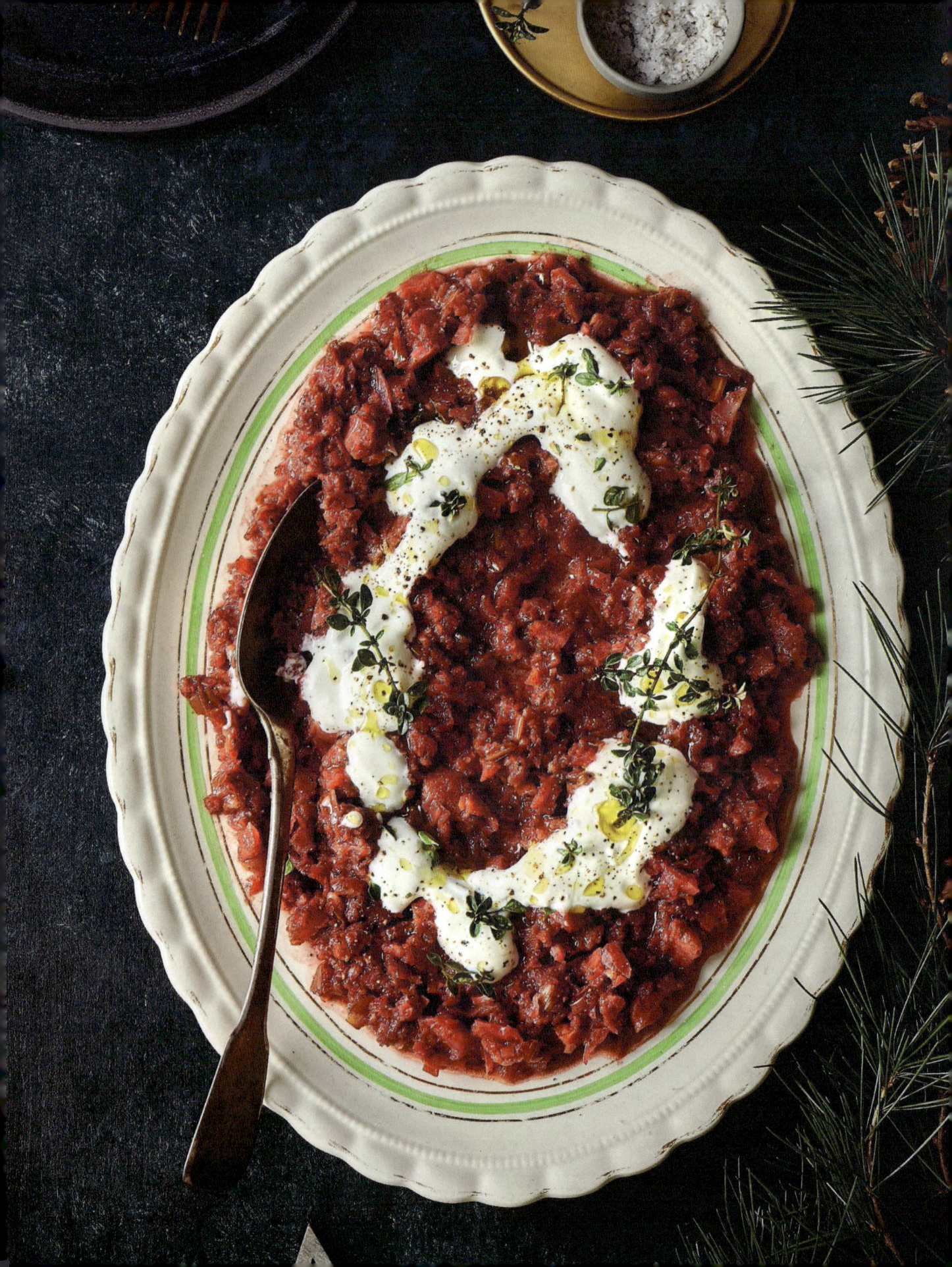

Beetroot & Red Wine Risotto with Goat's Cheese Cream

This deep red risotto has a wonderfully festive feel and an earthy, sweet flavour contrasting against the silky goat's cheese cream. Making a risotto from Cauliflower rice is great for everyone, carb intolerant or not. Once you get the hang of using cauli rice rather than the traditional Arborio, you can easily swap the additions according to the seasons.

Serves 4

100g (3½oz) butter
1 medium leek, finely chopped
3 teaspoons thyme leaves, plus a little extra to serve
300g (10 ½ oz) raw or cooked beetroot (not in vinegar)
600g (1lb 5oz) cauliflower, riced
1 teaspoon salt
plenty of freshly ground black pepper
150ml (5fl oz) red wine
50g Parmesan or other hard cheese, grated
150g (5½oz) soft, spreadable goat's cheese
extra virgin olive or truffle oil, to serve

Heat the butter in a large, heavy-based frying pan over a medium heat. Sauté the leek and thyme with seasoning for 10 minutes or until the leek is soft.

Meanwhile, purée the beetroot with 300ml (10 ½ fl oz) water in a food processor or with a stick blender until smooth and set aside.

Add the cauliflower rice to the pan with the seasoning and continue to fry for 5 minutes. Add the red wine, puréed beetroot and continue to cook, stirring all the time for a further 5 minutes. Bring to the boil and cook over a medium heat for 7 – 10 minutes or until the cauliflower is soft and tender. If the risotto looks dry, loosen it with a splash of hot water to create a creamy consistency.

To make the goat's cheese cream, use a fork to whisk the cheese in a small bowl with a tablespoon of cold water. If it is still very thick, add a little more water. You should have a light, whipped cream that drops easily from a spoon.

Add the Parmesan then taste the risotto and adjust the seasoning as necessary. Spoon it into warm bowls, spoon over the goat's cheese cream, add a swirl of oil, scatter over the thyme and give it a twist of black pepper.

Per serving: 19g net carbs, 4.8g fibre, 18g protein, 38g fat, 520kcal

Get ahead: Unlike a regular risotto, cauliflower rice risotto can be made in advance and reheated as you need in a pan on the hob or in the microwave.

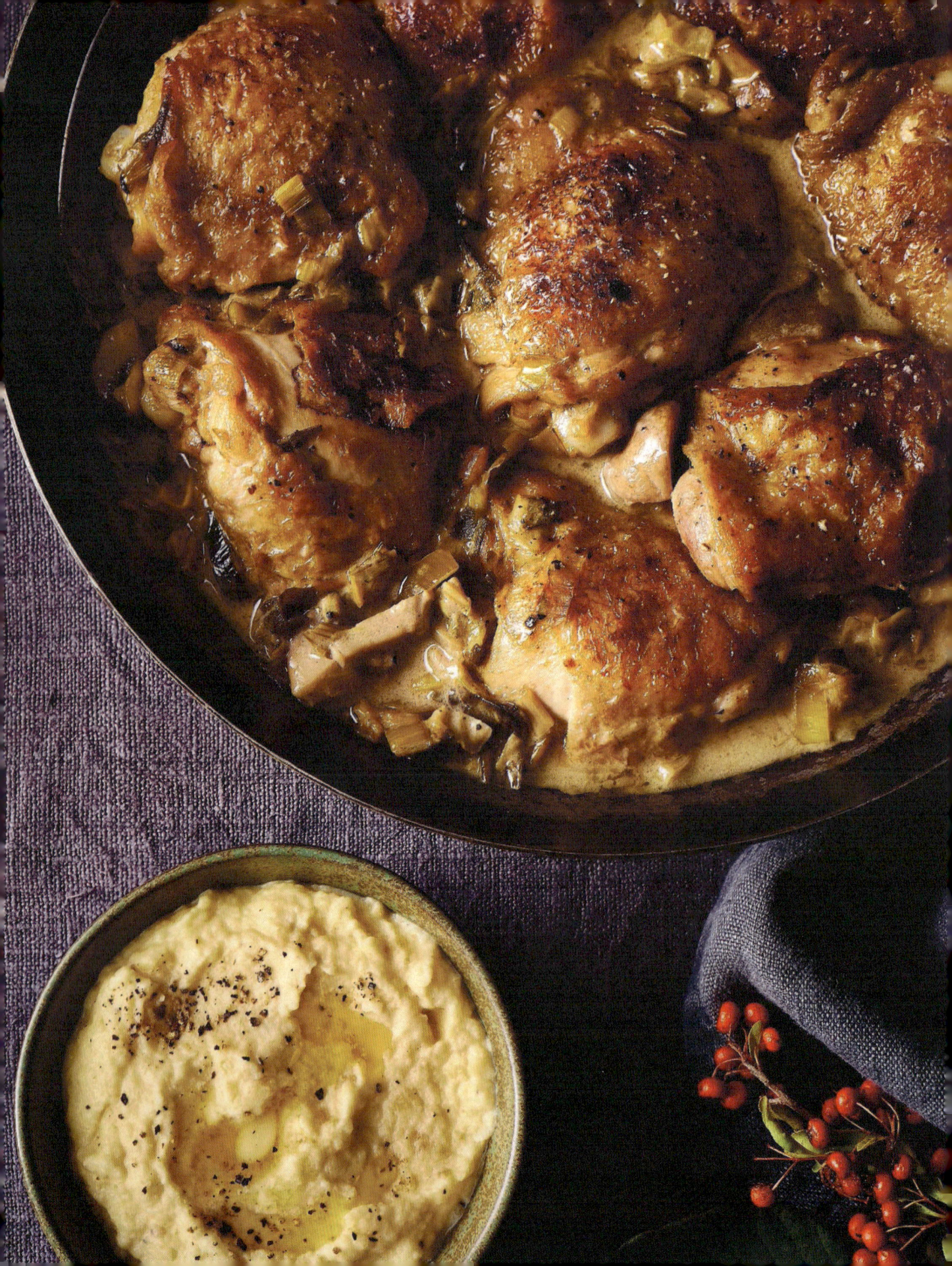

Chicken Thighs with Sage & Leek Cream Sauce

For the nutritional analysis I have allowed 2 chicken thighs per person but depending on their size you may find one each is enough for some. In the photograph we have shown this with the [Mashed Swede](#) which is our favourite side to have with it but you could also try the [Roasties.](#) The dried porcini enrich the mushroom flavour and give an umami hit to the recipe but omit them if you don't have them in.

Serves 4

10g (¼oz) dried porcini mushrooms
8 medium chicken thighs, skin on
25g (1oz) butter
1 medium leek, finely sliced
250g (9oz) small chestnut or button mushrooms, halved
16 broad sage leaves, roughly chopped
150ml (5fl oz) dry white wine
100ml (3½fl oz) double cream
salt and freshly ground black pepper

Cover the porcini mushrooms with 50ml (2fl oz) warm water and leave to soak while you cook the chicken.

Fry the chicken thighs in a large, non-stick frying pan, skin-side down, for about 20 minutes or until rich golden brown. They will release fat from the skin as they cook. Season the chicken in the pan and turn when browned. Cook for a further 15 minutes or so until golden brown. Transfer the chicken to a roasting tray and set aside.

If you have a lot of oil in the pan, tip some into a heatproof bowl to use another day, leaving a couple of tablespoons in the pan. Add the butter to the pan and set over a medium-high heat. When the butter is foaming, add the leek and mushrooms and stir-fry for about 15 minutes.

Drain the porcini mushrooms through a sieve and discard the water. Add these to the pan with the sage and stir through. Add the chicken back into the pan, skin-side up. Pour in the wine and bring to the boil. Reduce the wine for 5 minutes, then add the cream and once bubbling, reduce the heat to medium and let the chicken slowly bubble for about 20 minutes or until cooked through and falling off the bones. Serve straight away.

Per serving: 4.8g net carbs, 1.3g fibre, 48.6g protein, 39.1g fat, 602kcal

Get ahead: The chicken can be cooled and kept in the fridge for 3 days or frozen. Defrost thoroughly before reheating to piping hot.

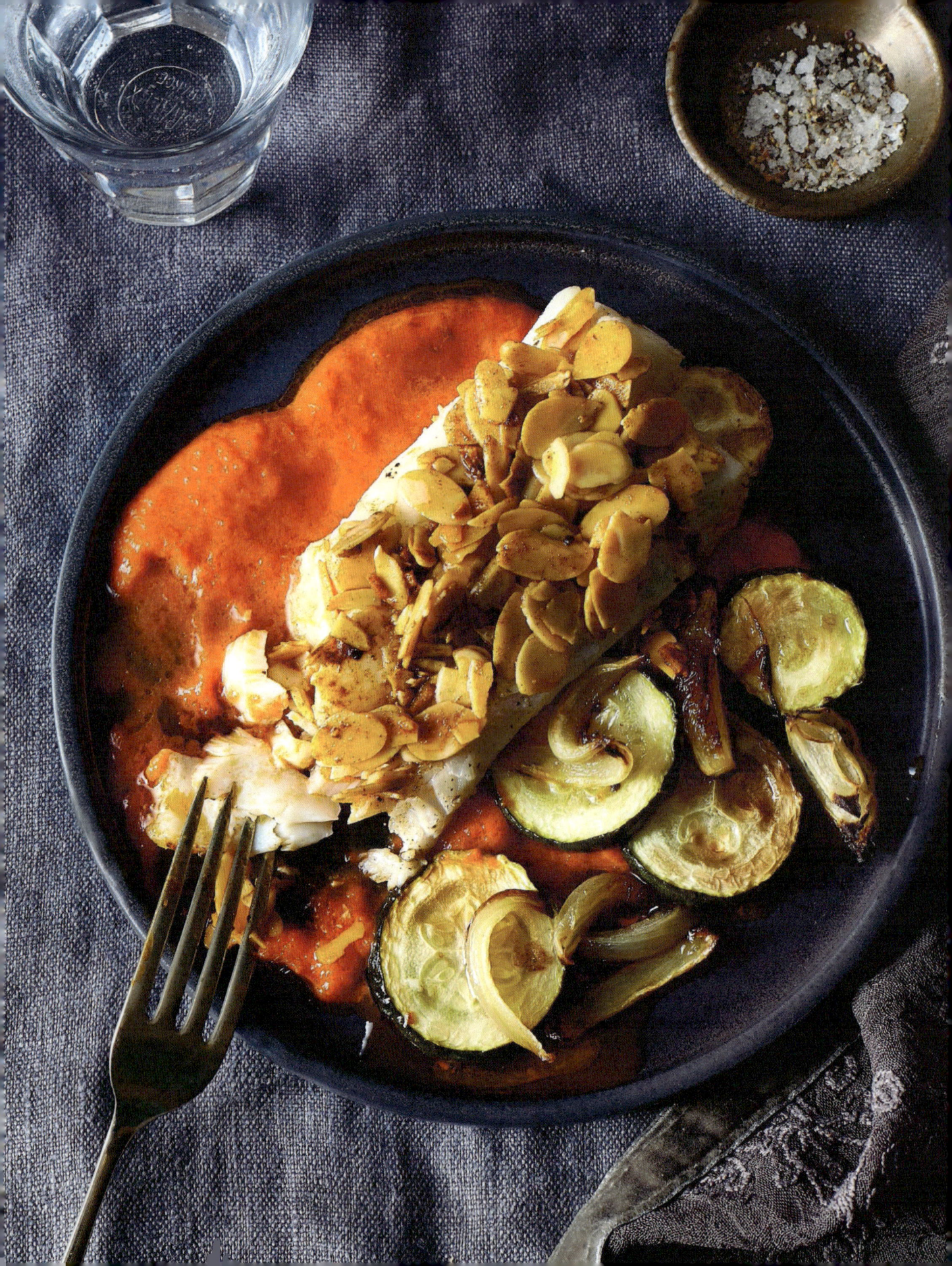

Baked Fish with Red Pepper Sauce & Spicy Almonds on Roast Vegetables

This smoky rich red sauce is extremely versatile and keeps well for a few days in the fridge. Make a batch and use it with roast vegetables, boiled eggs, grilled halloumi or sausages.

Serves 4

1 courgette, cut into 1cm (½in) slices
1 onion, cut into 2cm (¾in) wedges
2 tablespoons extra virgin olive oil
25g (1oz) butter
1 fat garlic clove, finely chopped
2 teaspoons smoked paprika
50g (1 ¾ oz) flaked almonds
4 fillets of hake, cod, halibut or similar white fish, skinned (approx. 600g/1lb 5oz)
salt and freshly ground black pepper

For the red pepper sauce

2 large red (bell) peppers
2 tablespoons extra virgin olive oil
salt, to taste

Preheat the oven to 220°C/200°C fan/400°F/gas mark 6.

Roast the peppers on a baking tray for 40 minutes or until blackened and blistered all over. Remove them from the oven and leave to cool in a bowl covered with a cloth. When cool enough to handle, pull off the skin and discard the seeds and core. Blitz the peppers into a purée with the oil and salt to taste in a food processor or using a stick blender. Transfer the sauce into a small saucepan.

Scatter the courgette and onion over a baking tray and toss in the oil and some seasoning. Spread the vegetables out into a single layer and roast for 15 minutes.

Meanwhile, heat the butter in a frying pan over a medium heat. Add the garlic, paprika, almonds and some seasoning and continue to fry until they are lightly browned. Remove from the heat.

Season the fish on both sides. Remove the baking tray from the oven and lay the fish on top of the vegetables. Return to the oven and cook for 6–8 minutes or until the fish is opaque all the way through; this will depend on the thickness of the fish.

Heat the pepper sauce over a low heat. When the fish is cooked, remove the tray from the oven. Spoon a little sauce over each plate. Divide the fish and vegetables between the plates and top each piece of fish with some spicy almonds. Serve straight away.

Per serving: 8.3g net carbs, 4.6g fibre, 29g protein, 27g fat, 397kcal
Get ahead: Make the pepper sauce a couple of days ahead and keep it in the fridge. Have the almond topping ready in the pan and warm through as the fish cooks.

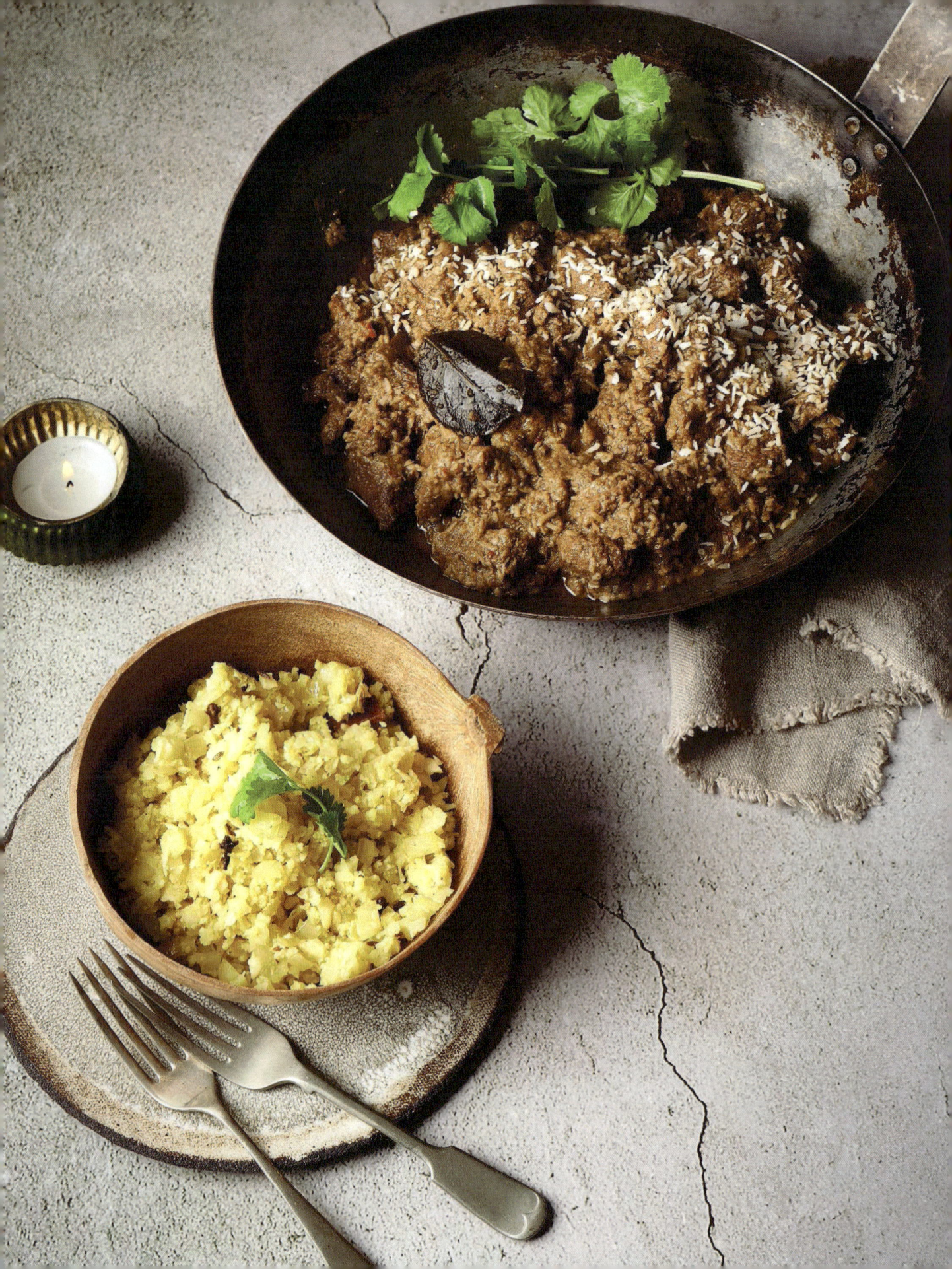

Malaysian Beef Rendang

Beef Rendang is a traditional Malaysian dish bursting with flavour from cardamon, star anise and lemongrass with natural sweetness from the coconut. We learned this dish about 15 years ago from chef and friend Caroline Milli Artiss and have been making it ever since with a few twists of our own. You can use a muslin bag for the spices or pick them out as you see them. The curry lasts well so I often double the quantities. It is lovely with [cauli rice.](#)

Serves 6

For the curry
75g (2½oz) desiccated coconut
2 tablespoons coconut or extra virgin olive oil
6 cloves
8 cardamom pods
5 star anise
2 small cinnamon sticks
1kg (2lb 4oz) beef (topside or stewing steak is fine), cubed
1 tablespoon tamarind paste or juice of ½ lemon
1 lemongrass stalk, crushed at the end
4 lime leaves
400ml (14fl oz) coconut milk
2 tablespoons tamari or dark gluten-free soy sauce
coriander leaves, to serve

For the spice paste
75g (2½oz) piece of fresh ginger, peeled
3 fresh hot chillies or 1 teaspoon chilli flakes
1 medium onion, quartered
4 fat garlic cloves
2 lemongrass stalks, outer layer removed

Dry-fry the coconut in a pan, stirring constantly until it turns brown and smells fantastic. Leave in a bowl to cool for later.

Put all the spice paste ingredients in a blender and with 2 tablespoons of water and blitz until it turns into paste.

Heat the oil in a large saucepan and add the spice paste, cloves, cardamom, star anise and cinnamon sticks and gently fry for about 5 minutes. Add the beef, tamarind, crushed lemongrass and lime leaves and fry until the beef turns brown, then add the coconut milk. Bring to the boil and then reduce the heat to its lowest setting and cover the pan. Cook for 1 hour, checking every now and then to make sure there is still some liquid and it is not sticking to the bottom of the pan. If it starts to look dry, add a little water.

After an hour, remove the lid and leave to simmer for a further 30 minutes. This is meant to be a dry dish so this will let the liquid evaporate a little. When the beef is tender and falling apart it is ready, then add the toasted coconut (reserving a tablespoon to serve) and soy sauce and stir together. Taste and adjust the seasoning with salt if necessary. Serve straight away with the cauli rice.

Per serving: 7.7g net carbs, 2.5g fibre, 40.7g protein, 56.2g fat, 713kcal
Get ahead: Cool the curry to room temperature and store in the fridge for up to 5 days or freeze for up to 3 months.

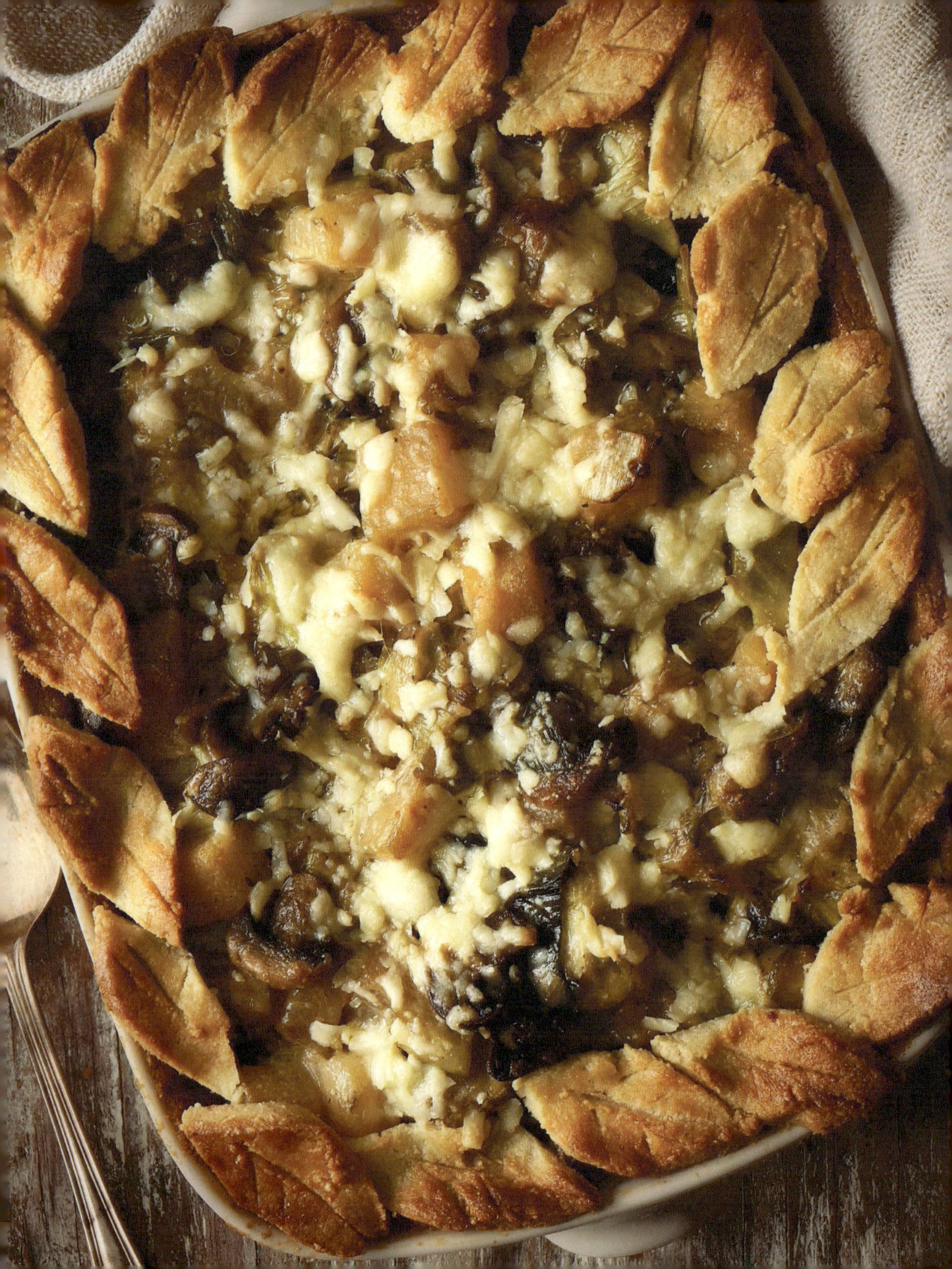

Homity Pie

Leftover cooked vegetables were transformed into dinner during the second world war by the LandGirls and so Homity Pie was born. It was made famous by the vegetarian restaurant group Cranks in the 1970s and is still a great way to use up leftovers from a roast dinner. Add what you like in place of the leek, swede and mushrooms, including leftover cooked meat, as long as you have about 1.3kg (3lb) in weight to fill the pie. We like to add truffle oil to our sauce for a Christmas indulgence but at other times a spoonful of thyme leaves adds a wonderful flavour.

Serves 8
For the filling

50g (1¾oz) butter, plus a little for greasing
1 large leek, approx. 400g (14oz), cut into finger width slices
500g (1lb 2oz) swede, peeled and cut into 2cm (¾in) dice
400g (7oz) small button mushrooms, roughly sliced
4–5 teaspoons truffle oil or 1 teaspoon thyme leaves
1 fat garlic clove, finely chopped
250ml (9fl oz) double cream
100g (3½oz) mature Cheddar or other hard cheese, finely grated
salt and freshly ground black pepper

For the pastry
1 medium egg, beaten
150g (5½oz) cold salted butter, cut into small cubes
200g (7oz) ground almonds
30g (1oz) coconut flour

To make the pastry divide the beaten egg mixture in half and reserve half in a small bowl to brush the pie before cooking. Mix the other half with the remaining pastry ingredients in a mixing bowl using a spatula or spoon. Transfer the pastry on to a piece of baking parchment, wrap and chill in the fridge.

Preheat the oven to 180°C fan/200°C/400°F/gas mark 6 and grease a pie dish measuring about 25 x 20cm (10 x 8in) with butter.

To make the filling, heat the butter in a large frying pan over a medium heat and fry the vegetables, thyme, if using, and garlic with seasoning, stirring occasionally, for 15–20 minutes until just soft. Add the cream and half the Cheddar. Taste the vegetables and add more seasoning and the truffle oil, if using, to taste. Remove from the heat.

Roll out the pastry between two sheets of baking parchment to 5mm (¼in). Line the bottom of the pie dish, trimming off the edges. Save the trimmings for making the leaves; wrap them in parchment and put in the fridge. Prick the base a few times with a fork. Blind bake the pie crust by covering the pastry with one of the pieces of baking parchment. Fill the pie with rice or beans (this will help to keep the pastry in place). Bake for 10 minutes. Carefully tip out the rice to cool and use again another day. Remove the parchment and put the pie back in the oven for 2 minutes to firm up the base.

Fill the pie with the filling and scatter over the remaining Cheddar. Roll out the pastry trimmings and cut into leaf shapes. Gently press these onto the edges of the pie and brush with the remaining beaten egg. Bake for 15 minutes or until the pastry is golden brown. Drizzle a swirl of truffle oil, if using, on top just before serving to boost the aroma and serve straight away.

Per serving made with truffle oil: 12.7g net carbs, 7.3g fibre, 16.9g protein, 75g fat, 810kcal

Get ahead: The pie crust can be made in advance to the point that it has been blind-baked, cooled and kept for up to a day in the fridge. The filling can also be made in ahead of time and warmed through before filling the pie. The leaves can be shaped and kept in the fridge. So, all you have to do is fill the pie, finish it with the Cheddar, pastry leaves and egg wash and bake for 15 minutes or until hot and golden brown.

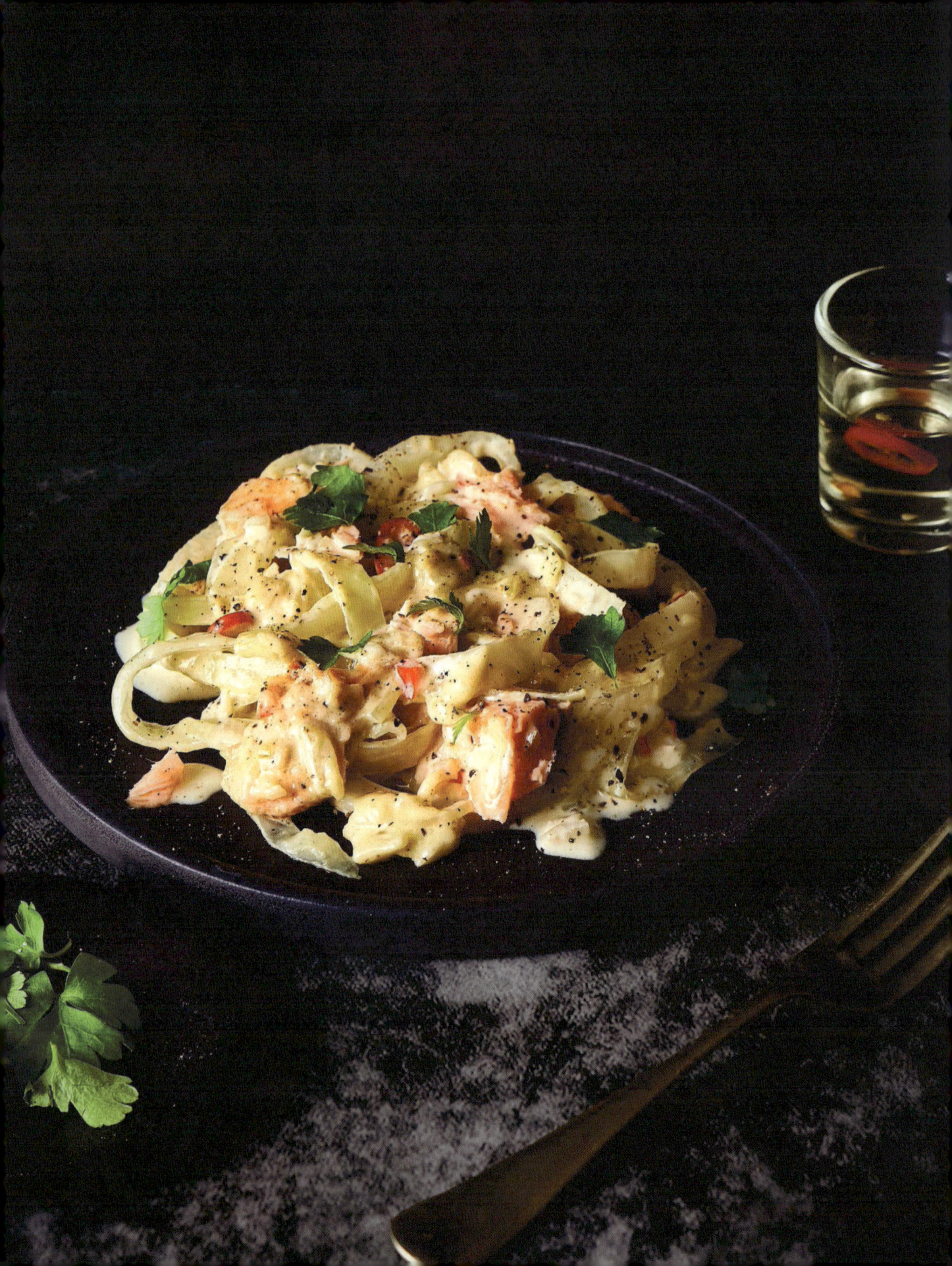

Creamy hot smoked salmon on cabbage pasta ribbons with chilli vodka

Let's have some Christmas fun! This is a winter warmer that we serve with shots of chilli vodka – it adds a real kick and a giggle to the meal. You can make your own chilli vodka by adding a whole hot red chilli to a bottle of vodka and leaving it for at least 4 days. You can leave it there forever and the vodka will become spicier as time goes by and do try it in the [Smoky Mary.](#) Hot-smoked salmon is cooked and smoked at the same time, it has a gentle taste of smoke. If you can't find it, use half the amount of smoked salmon instead. Soft ribbons of white cabbage are a really good alternative to traditional tagliatelle or fettucine pasta. Any cabbage will do, from earthy cavolo nero to bright green Savoy, each bringing their own colour, texture and flavour. White cabbage is slightly sweet and firmer, so it takes a couple of minutes more cooking to transform it into soft, tender ribbons. Cabbage pasta ribbons are excellent with any pasta sauce from Bolognese to tomato and cheese. Do taste your chilli for heat before adding it – the heat is in the pith so try it for strength in the middle, not the ends. Seeds can be left in or out.

Serves 4

For the sauce

2 tablespoons extra virgin olive oil
1 garlic clove, finely chopped
6 tablespoons chilli or normal vodka (see intro)
360g (12 ½ oz) hot-smoked salmon
250ml (9 fl oz) double cream
roughly chopped fresh parsley, to serve
1 white onion, finely chopped
1 red or green hot chilli, finely sliced, added according to strength or ½ teaspoon chilli flakes

For the cabbage pasta ribbons

½ head of white or savoy cabbage (approx. 500–700g/1lb 2oz–1lb 9oz)
10g (¼oz) salted butter
salt and freshly ground black pepper

Divide the cabbage in half, remove the hard core or stems and outer raggedy leaves. Lay the cabbage flat side down and use a sharp knife to cut it into 1cm (½in) ribbons.

Pull the ribbons apart and put them into a medium saucepan with the butter, 100ml (3½fl oz) water and some salt and pepper, and cover with a lid. Cook over a medium heat for 8–10 minutes or until the ribbons are very soft and tender.

Meanwhile, make the sauce. Fry the onion, chilli and garlic in the olive oil in a large frying pan over a medium heat for about 5 minutes until soft but not coloured. Add salt and a generous amount of black pepper. Pour in the chilli vodka and ignite if you wish (stand back) or simply leave for a couple of minutes to burn off the alcohol. Flake the salmon into the pan and pour in the cream. Cook briefly over a low heat for a couple of minutes to thicken the sauce.

Add the cabbage and any cooking juices to the pan with the salmon and cream. Toss through gently so as not to break up the salmon. Taste and adjust the seasoning and heat from the chilli accordingly. Divide between warm bowls and serve with a sprinkling of fresh parsley.

Per serving of cabbage: 7.5g net carbs, 1.8g protein, 2.2g fat, 4.5g fibre, 66kcal
Per serving of cabbage and sauce: 9.4 net carbs, 3.8g fibre, 24.6g protein, 53.3g fat, 664kcal
Get ahead: Make your own chilli vodka in the few weeks before Christmas.

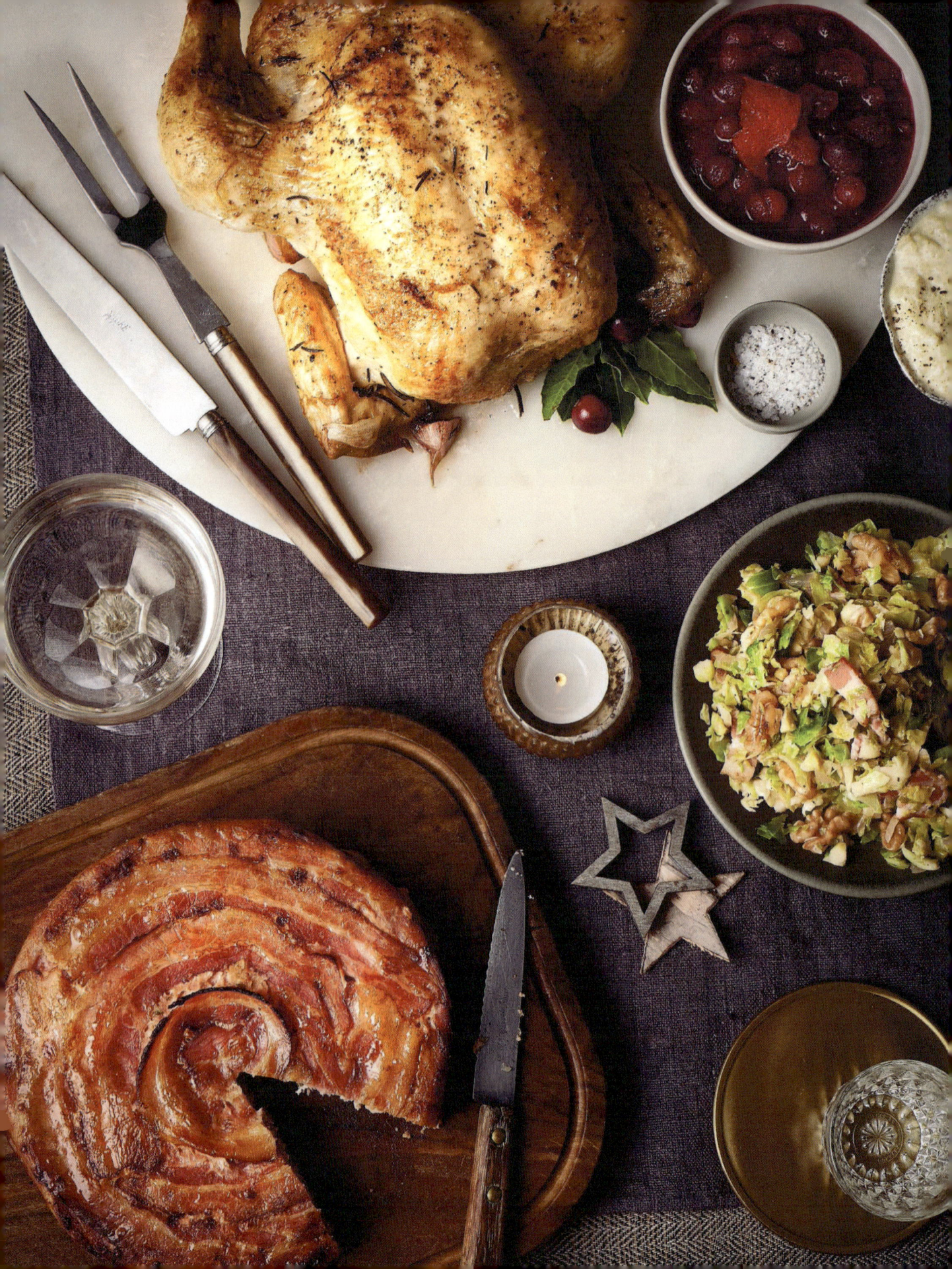

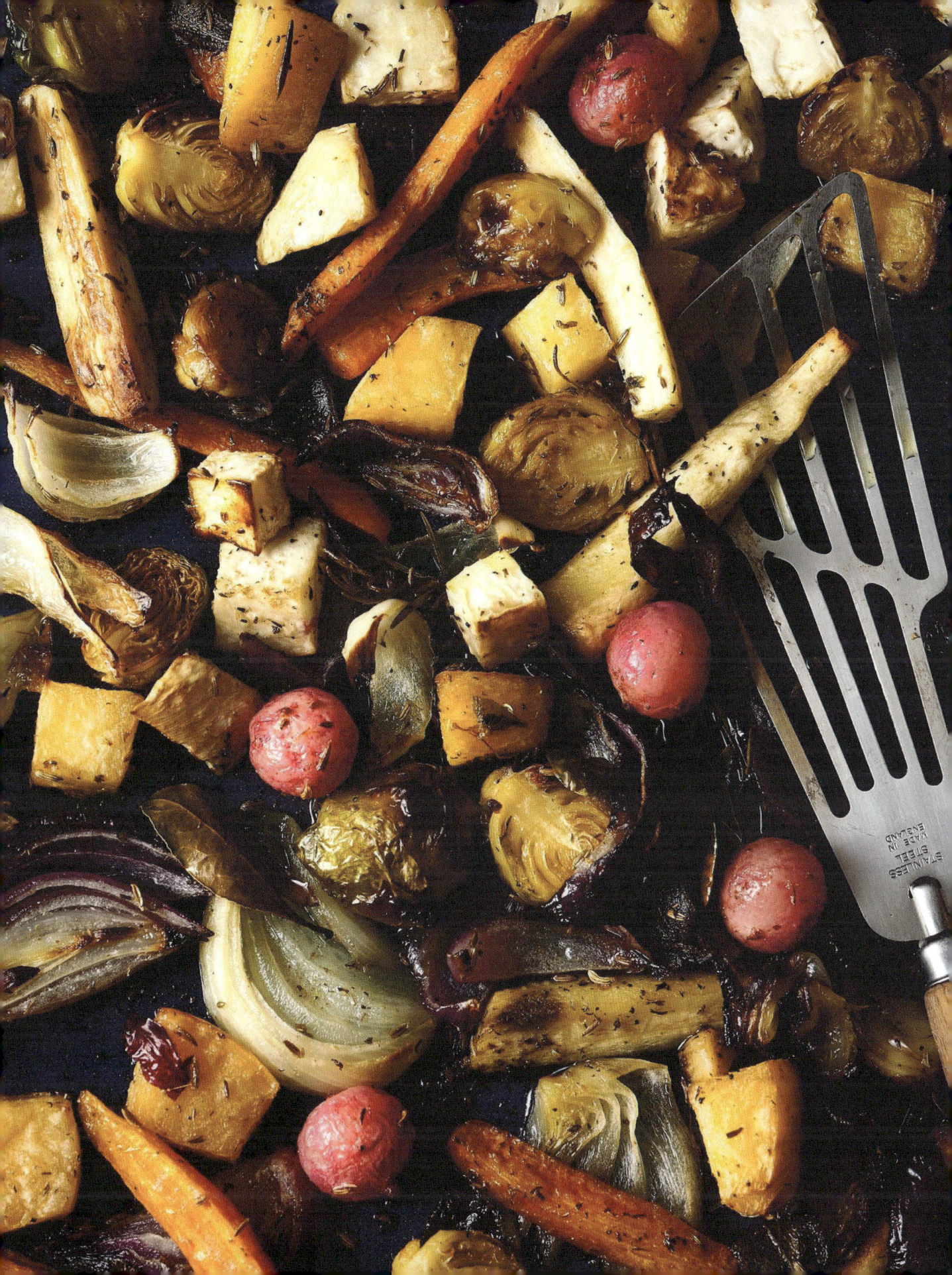

Side Dishes

I sometimes think low-carb cooking could be described as "how to eat more vegetables" as there are so many wonderful flavours to be enjoyed from using vegetable alternatives to carby potatoes or rice. Once you get to know the carb values of various vegetables, you can easily make swaps to keep your blood glucose in check. Think of swede rather than potato for mash, ribbons of cabbage instead of pappardelle, roasted vegetables or steamed broccoli as a base for a pasta sauce, [cauli rice](#) instead of white rice or celeriac instead of potato in a [dauphinoise.](#)

Sage & Onion Stuffing Cake

For this recipe, it's best to use thin streaky bacon as it bends easily into a spiral. You can make it without the [cauliflower rice,](#) but I found that, like breadcrumbs, the rice softens the pork and adds moisture to stop it becoming dry. The cake can be prepared in advance and kept in the fridge until you are ready to cook it. Any leftovers can be reheated in foil in the oven or microwave.

Serves 6

10g (¼oz) butter
200g (7oz) thin rashers of smoked streaky bacon
1 medium onion, finely chopped
100g (3½oz) [cauli rice](#)
500g (1lb 2oz) pork mince
1 apple, finely chopped
2 tablespoons fresh sage, finely chopped or 1 tablespoon dried sage
2 medium eggs
½ teaspoon salt
plenty of freshly ground black pepper

Butter a 20cm (8in) loose-bottomed cake tin. Use the bacon to line the dish in a spiral, starting in the centre. When you reach the edges of the base, push the rashers up slightly to form a corner to seal in the pork. Wind the bacon around the sides too. If you have any left over, chop it finely and put it into a bowl.

Preheat the oven to 200°C/180°C fan/400°F/gas mark 6.

Mix the remaining ingredients together thoroughly in the bowl with the any leftover bacon. Now pack the mixture into the bacon-lined tin being careful not to dislodge the rashers.

Bake the stuffing for 30 minutes or until firm to the touch and cooked through. Remove from the oven and take out of the tin. Wipe away any juices that have leaked out of the meat. Return the cake to the oven for 15–20 minutes to brown. Serve straight away or keep it warm for up to 30 minutes before serving.

Per serving: 5.6g net carbs, 1.3g fibre, 24.3g protein, 14.9g fat, 256kcal

Get ahead: Make the cake up to 2 days before serving, then bring to room temperature for 30 minutes before cooking as above.

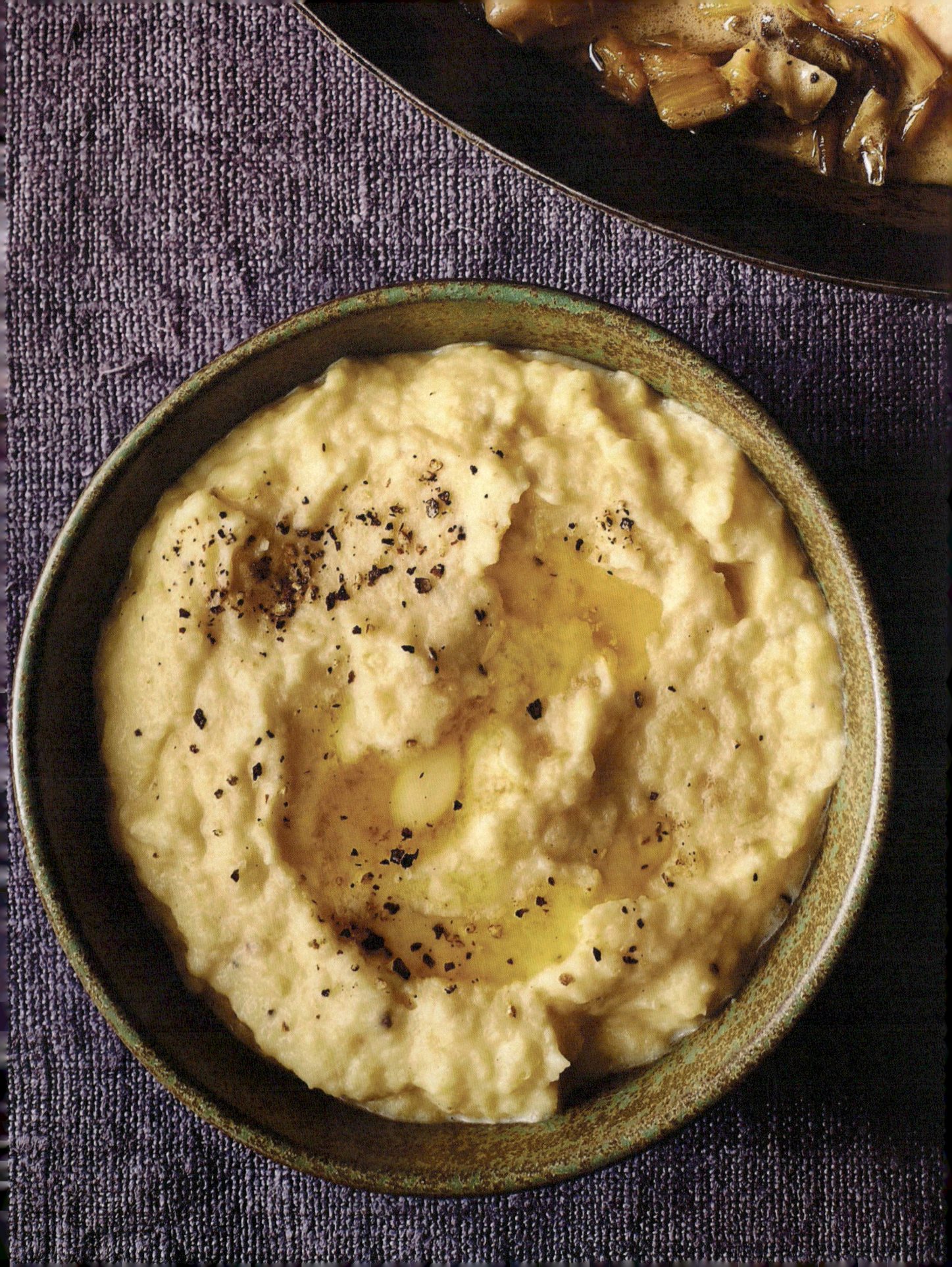

Mashed Swede

This pale orange mash is delicately spicy and slightly sweet. It makes a creamy contrast to any main course and any leftovers are wonderful with bacon and eggs.

Serves 6

400g (14oz) swede, diced roughly into approx. 3cm (1¼in) cubes
50g (1¾oz) butter
100ml (3½fl oz) double cream
½ teaspoon nutmeg (optional)
salt and freshly ground black pepper

Boil the swede in salted water for 25–30 minutes until tender.

Drain the swede through a colander and put it into a food processor to blend or back into the pan and use a potato masher. Add the remaining ingredients and blend again until smooth. Taste and adjust the seasoning as necessary. Serve straight away or put into a serving dish and keep warm.

Per serving: 1.8g net carbs, 0.5g fibre, 0.5g protein, 15.3g fat, 143kcal

Get ahead: The mash can be made in advanced and reheated in a pan. If it is too thick, let it down with a little cream or milk.

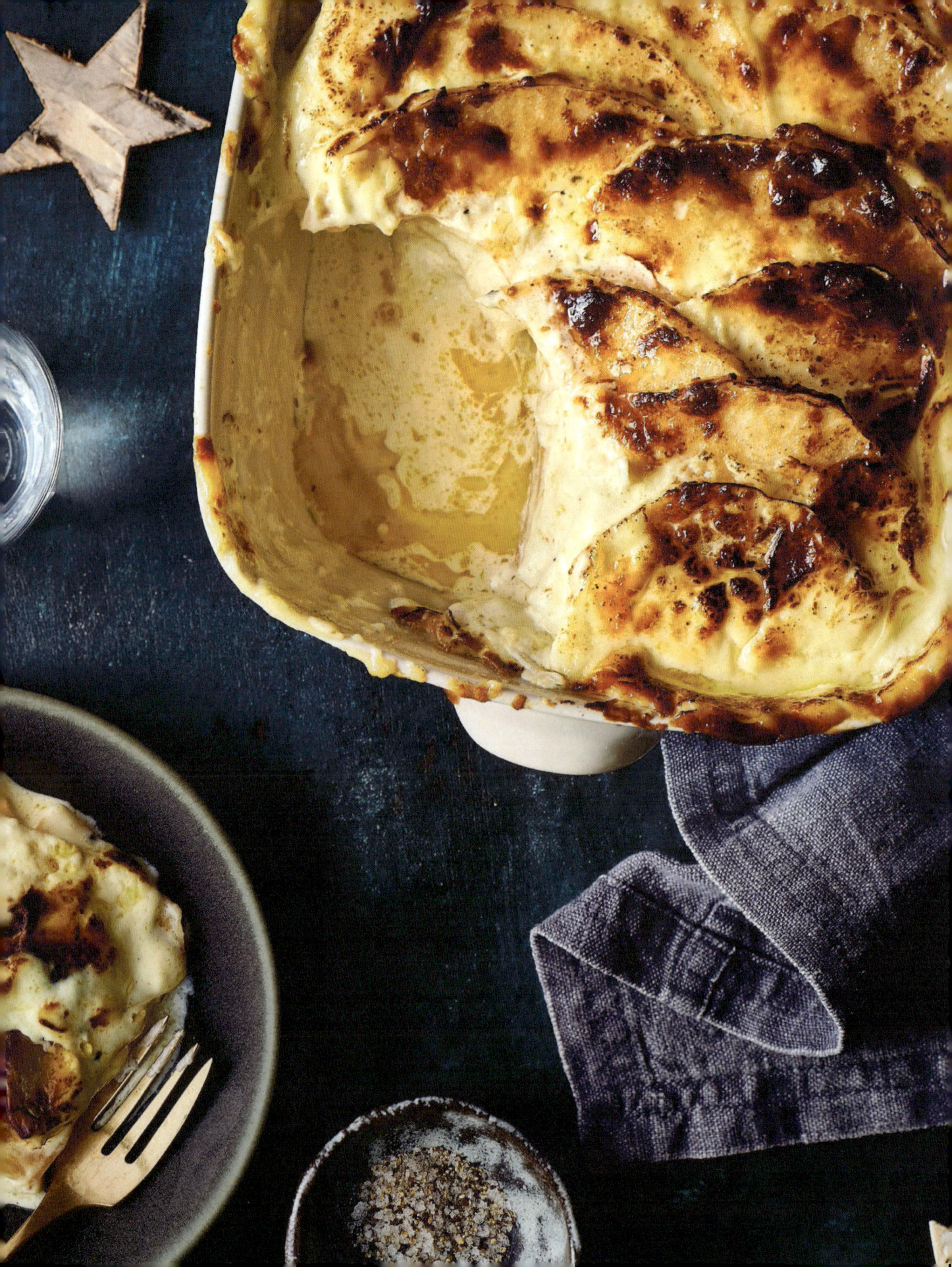

Celeriac & Swede Dauphinoise

You will get far more flavour and less carbs from using root vegetables, such as celeriac, swede or turnips, instead of potatoes. Use one or enjoy a mixture of them together. This dish takes a while to cook so it's great to bake while you have a roast in the oven. It is high in calories as a side but for a treat, it is delicious. Try leftovers it with a couple of poached eggs and bacon for lunch.

Serves 8

600ml (20fl oz) double cream
3 fat garlic cloves, finely chopped
½ teaspoon grated nutmeg
100g (3 ½ fl oz) butter, melted
800g–1kg (1lb 12oz–2lb 4oz) celeriac and/or swede, peeled and finely sliced
50g (1 ¾ oz) Gruyère or Parmesan cheese, finely grated
salt and freshly ground black pepper

Preheat the oven to 200°C/180°C fan/400°F/gas mark 6.

Mix the cream, garlic, nutmeg, butter and seasoning together in a bowl.

Put a layer of celeriac into an ovenproof dish – we use a round one 25cm (10in) in diameter and about 6cm (2½in) deep, but any similar sized dish will work. Pour over a layer of the cream followed by a little cheese. Repeat this until both the ingredients are used up, finishing with the cheese.

Cover with foil to avoid it drying out and bake for 1½ hours. Remove the foil and let it brown for a further 20–30 minutes or until the vegetables are tender when pierced with a knife. Leave to stand for 10 minutes before serving.

Per serving: 6.4g net carbs, 0.9g fibre, 4.1g protein, 50.3g fat, 487kcal

Get ahead: This can be baked in advanced and reheated in a hot oven under foil or put into the microwave, uncovered. It will keep before cooking in the fridge for up to a day and leftovers keep for four days in the fridge. It can be frozen at any stage for up to 3 months.

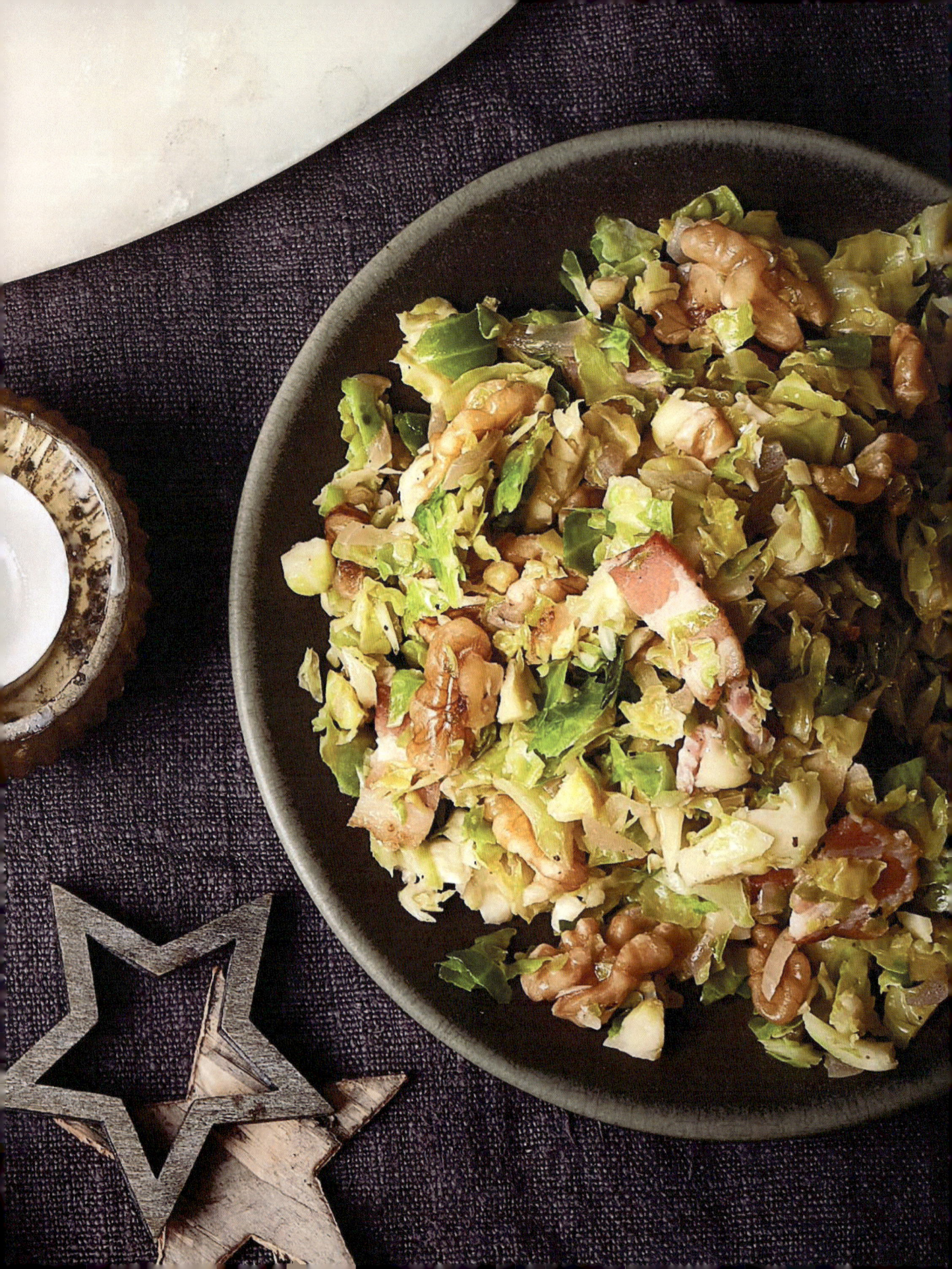

Stir-fried Sprouts with Onion, Bacon & Walnuts

Use whole sprouts – I never peel or trim them unless the leaves are damaged or soft. Chestnuts are higher in carbs than other nuts, so I have replaced them with soaked walnuts or pecans to offer a creamy texture and golden colour. These sprouts are so tasty that they make a good meal on their own or with a couple of fried eggs.

Serves 6

75g (2½oz) walnuts or pecans
1 tablespoon extra-virgin olive oil
25g (1oz) butter
1 onion, finely chopped
4 thick rashers of smoked streaky bacon, cut into strips
500g (1lb 2oz) Brussels sprouts
salt and freshly ground black pepper

Put the nuts into a small bowl with just-boiled water to soak.

Fry the onion and bacon together in the oil and butter in a large frying pan or wok over a medium heat. Season lightly.

Shred the sprouts in a food processor or cut them by hand. Once the bacon is cooked and the onions are translucent, add the sprouts and drained nuts to the pan with 100ml (3½fl oz) water. Stir-fry them over a high heat to mingle the flavours. Cover with a lid, increase the heat to medium and cook for 5 minutes, shaking the pan occasionally.

Remove the lid and check that they are just soft. If not, fry for a little longer. Taste and adjust the seasoning as necessary. Serve straight away, keep warm in an open serving bowl in a warm place or keep them in the pan and finish cooking just before serving.

Per serving: 6.1g net carbs, 3.3g fibre, 7.3g protein, 18.7g fat, 220kcal

Get ahead: You can fry the bacon and onion and have them ready in a pan. Shred the sprouts and keep them in an airtight container in the fridge.

Roasties

We love the jewel-like colours of these roast vegetables and the flavour from the herbs is fantastic. You won't miss potatoes at all! All of the peelings can be kept in the freezer and used for a homemade stock another day.

Serves 6

1kg (2lb 4oz) root vegetables such as carrots, parsnip, celeriac, swede, radishes, Brussels sprouts or turnips
5 tablespoons extra virgin olive oil
1 onion, cut into wedges
4 small sprigs of rosemary
1 teaspoon dried oregano
4 bay leaves
6 large sage leaves, roughly chopped
2 teaspoons fennel seeds
2 fat garlic cloves, unpeeled and crushed
salt and freshly ground black pepper

Preheat the oven to 220°C/200°C fan/425°F/gas mark 7.

Scrub and cut the carrots and parsnips, if using, into wedges that are about 3cm (1¼in) at the fattest end. Peel and dice the swede and/or celeriac into 3cm (1¼in) dice and cut the sprouts in half. Toss the vegetables in a bowl with the oil, seasoning, herbs and spices. Spread them out on a baking tray and roast for 30 minutes or until cooked through. Serve straight away or keep warm, loosely covered, for up to 1 hour.

Per serving: 11.6g net carbs, 5.6g fibre, 1.2g protein, 11.8g fat, 168kcal

Get ahead: The roasties are best served straight from the oven but can be prepared to the point just before cooking and kept in a bowl in the fridge for up to a day. Leftovers can be reheated under foil in the oven until piping hot or used in the Homity Pie.

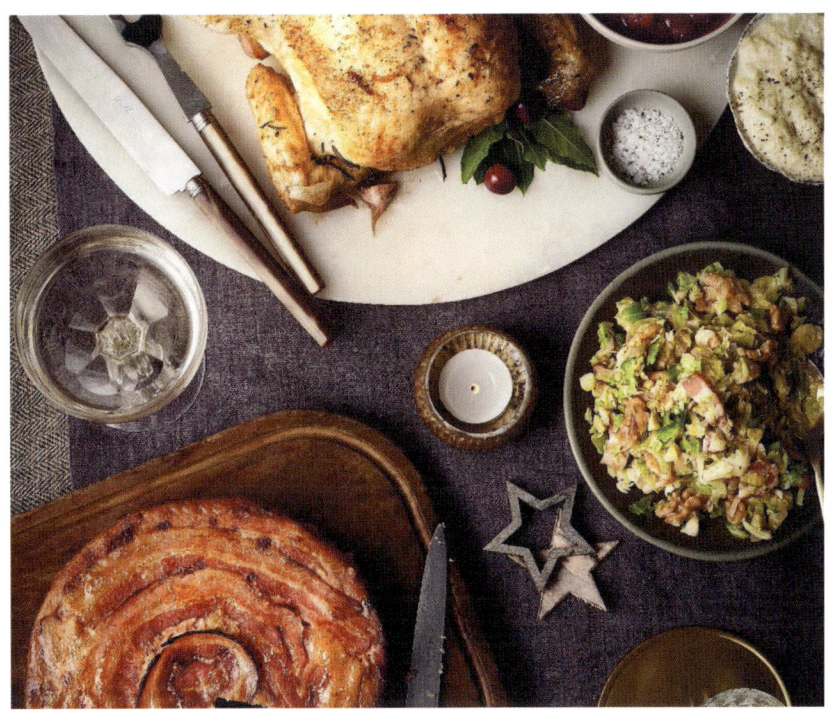

Cranberry Sauce

Cranberries are naturally sour in flavour. If you are a hardened no-sugar person, you may find the sweetness of the orange is enough for you. For others the sourness can be adjusted with minimal honey or erythritol.

Serves 8

300g (10½oz) cranberries
3 long peelings from an orange, plus juice of 1 orange
1 tablespoon honey or 2 tablespoons erythritol
100ml (3½fl oz) dry white wine

Put all the ingredients into a saucepan and bring to the boil. Reduce the heat so that the mixture bubbles gently and continue to cook, stirring frequently, until the berries begin to burst. At this point taste the sauce for sweetness and adjust accordingly. Remove from the heat and leave to cool before serving.

Per serving: 6.4g net carbs, 1.4g fibre, 0.3g protein, 0.1g fat, 39kcal
Per serving without honey: 4.3g net carbs, 1.4g fibre, 0.3g protein, 0.1g fat, 31kcal

Get ahead: The sauce keeps in the fridge for up to a week or can be frozen.

"Bread" Sauce

This was always one of my favourite parts of Christmas lunch but when half the family were diagnosed as gluten-intolerant and then we all became low-carb, it seemed pointless to make it. Now I have discovered the joys of cauliflower in all its forms, it only took a small leap of faith to see if I could make it into "bread" sauce. I am happy to say it was a hit with the whole family and it is back on our festive table again. Almond milk is lower in carbs than cow's milk but either work.

Serves 8

1 small onion, halved
8 cloves
200g (7oz) [cauliflower, riced](#)
150ml (5fl oz) whole almond or cow's milk
50ml (2fl oz) double cream
1 bay leaf
10g (¼ oz) butter
salt and freshly ground black pepper

Stud half the onion with the cloves so they offer their flavour but don't become lost in the sauce. Put all the ingredients together in a medium saucepan and bring to the boil. Reduce the heat and simmer gently for 20–30 minutes or until the sauce has thickened. Stir occasionally to break up the cauliflower. Adjust the seasoning, then pick out the bay leaf and onion. Serve straight away.

Per serving: 1.8g net carbs, 0.7g fibre, 0.8g protein, 3.5g fat, 42kcal

Get ahead: Cool the sauce and keep in the fridge for up to 5 days.

The Gravy

A delicious gravy that can be made ahead of time. One thing I have realized over the years is that any leftover gravy makes a homemade soup come alive, so do freeze any for a soup day.

Makes approx. 600ml (20fl oz)/Serves 12

2 carrots, roughly chopped
2 onions, roughly chopped
2 celery sticks, roughly chopped
100g (3½oz) smoked or unsmoked bacon lardons or chopped streaky bacon
2 bay leaves
2 sprigs of rosemary or sage
8 chicken wings
2 tablespoons extra virgin olive oil
250ml (9fl oz) dry white wine
2 tablespoons cornflour (optional)
salt and freshly ground black pepper

Preheat the oven to 200°C/180°C fan/400°F/gas mark 6.

Put the vegetables into a roasting dish (that is suitable to heat on the hob later) and scatter over the bacon and herbs. Lay the wings over the top to protect the vegetables from burning and drizzle over the oil. Season lightly with salt and pepper.

Cook for 1½ hours or until the chicken is roasted to a golden brown but not burnt, see the photo. Remove the tray from the oven and transfer the chicken to a large saucepan.

Add 2 litres (3½ pints) of hot water from a kettle and bring to the boil. Reduce the heat to a gentle boil and simmer for 2 hours or until it has reduced by half. Use a potato masher to break up the chicken and crush the vegetables.

Strain the stock through a sieve, squeezing out as much flavour as possible from the chicken and vegetables with a wooden spoon.

Pour the liquid back into a saucepan and season to taste. If you prefer the gravy thicker, mix the cornflour with a splash of water in a bowl and add this to the gravy over the heat. Stir until thickened. The gravy is now ready to use – chill and store in the fridge or cool and freeze.

Per 50ml serving: 1.5g net carbs, 0.1g fibre, 0.1g protein, 2.3g fat, 41kcal

Get ahead: Keep the gravy in the fridge for 3 days and freeze for up to 3 months.

Cauliflower Rice

This is our favourite way to cook cauli rice. If only our local curry house sold it, I would be the first to order it – I'm sure it is only a matter of time. Until then I can make the rice in the time it takes for a curry to arrive, so I am not tempted to order white rice and naan. Broccoli rice can be made in the same way or use both vegetables mixed together. Add the leaves to the food processor too or cook them separately as [Cauli Crisps.](#)

Basic Cauliflower Rice

This is a simple way to prepare cauliflower rice and an excellent substitute for simple white rice.

Serves 6

800g–1kg (1lb 12oz–2lb 4oz) cauliflower (florets, stalk and leaves)
4 tablespoons extra virgin olive oil, ghee, coconut oil, chicken fat or beef dripping
1 onion, finely chopped, or 5 spring onions, finely chopped
1 teaspoon salt
freshly ground black pepper

Cut the head of the cauliflower into florets and roughly chop the stalk and leaves. Put one third of the cauliflower into a food processor and pulse until finely chopped (it will resemble large grains of rice), making sure you don't end up with a purée. Tip the cauliflower into a bowl and repeat with the remaining two thirds. Coarsely grate the florets and stalk and finely chop the leaves if you don't have a food processor.

Heat the oil or fat in a wok or large frying pan. Fry the onion over a medium heat for 7 minutes or until soft. Add the cauliflower rice, season and stir through. Cover and cook over a low heat for about 7 minutes or until just soft.

Indian Cauliflower Pilau

We love this with curries and add the traditional spices used to make pilau rice.

1 quantity of Basic Cauliflower Rice
1 teaspoon cumin seeds
5 cloves
5 cardamom pods, lightly crushed
2 bay leaves
1 small cinnamon stick
½ teaspoon ground turmeric
a few sprigs of coriander, roughly chopped

Follow the recipe for Basic [Cauliflower Rice](#), adding the spices to the onion once it is cooked. Scatter with coriander before serving.

Per serving of either cauli-rice: 3.9g net carbs, 2.2g fibre, 2g protein, 9.3g fat, 109kcal

Get ahead: Once cooked, this keeps well in the fridge for up to 3 days (or in the freezer for up to 3 months), so leftovers are quick to reheat.

Chapter Three

Bread, Pastry & Crackers

Low-carb baking means cooking without wheat and therefore not having any gluten in your bread or pastry. It takes a little getting used to but you soon become familiar with the alternatives such as flaxseed (also known as linseed), coconut flour and psyllium husk. You might see mozzarella used as a binder in place of gluten – as it's not really used for flavour, an inexpensive version is fine.

Flaxseed is either dark brown or golden; both are good to use so choose the colour you prefer. Pre-milled flaxseed is more expensive than buying the seeds and it is easy to grind your own in a small high-speed food processor. Do keep the seeds in the fridge or freezer as they can become rancid.

Psyllium husk is the outer shell of the seed of the Plantago ovata plant. In larger quantities it is used as a laxative as it is a form of insoluble fibre, but in baking it is used to absorb moisture and give structure. It comes as husks or powdered husks. The powder is more expensive so we use the husks. You can see our favourite brand in our shop at www.lowcarbtogether.com and make that a live link but not directly to the shop. When measured by weight it will be fine to use either, but if you see recipes with spoonfuls use slightly less of the powder.

You can see more baking tips on our website www.lowcarbtogether.com

Multi-Seed Crackers

We ate these seed-speckled crackers in Sweden where they were served with lashings of butter. Try flavouring the crackers with dried herbs, such as oregano or thyme, or seeds like onion, coriander, cumin or caraway. They keep well in an airtight container for up to 5 days.

Serves 8

extra virgin olive oil, to grease
150g (5 ½ oz) mixed seeds, such as sunflower, pumpkin, poppy, hemp, coriander, sesame
50g (1 ¾ oz) golden or dark flaxseed, ground
½ teaspoon fine salt
1 medium egg white (30g/1oz)
Preheat the oven to 200° C/fan 180° C/400 ° F/gas mark 6, line a baking tray with baking parchment and lightly brush it with oil.

Thoroughly mix the ingredients together in a large mixing bowl adding 5–6 tablespoons of cold water to form a thick paste. Use a spatula to scrape the mixture onto the prepared tray.

Take another piece of baking parchment the size of your baking tray and brush it with oil. Put this, oil-side down, on top of the mixture and use a short rolling pin or an empty wine bottle to roll it out until 2mm (1/16in) thick.

Remove the top piece of parchment and bake for 18–20 minutes or until lightly browned and brittle.

Once cool enough to touch, break the crackers into shards. If any of the crackers look undercooked underneath, simply put them back in the oven for a couple of minutes to crisp up.

Per 30g serving of crackers: 3g carbs, protein 6g, 11g fat, 2g fibre, 143kcal

Get ahead: Once the crackers are bone dry, they will keep in a paper bag at room temperature for a week.

Caraway & Walnut Baguettes

Way up high in the mountains on a skiing holiday to the Dolomites, I learned to cook a local bread packed with nuts, seeds and the mild, spicy taste of caraway. This is my low-carb, gluten-free version of that mountain bread. Do use an inexpensive cow's milk mozzarella, the sort you would use on pizza. We love this bread with butter and Cheddar cheese or try it thinly sliced and topped with cream cheese and smoked salmon.

Makes 4 small baguettes

75g (2½oz) dark flaxseed, ground
100g (3½oz) ground almonds
1 teaspoon gluten-free baking powder
1 teaspoon salt
100g (3½oz) walnuts, roughly chopped
50g (1¾oz) sunflower seeds
2 teaspoons caraway seeds (optional)
1 x 125g (4½oz) mozzarella ball, coarsely grated
50ml (2fl oz) mozzarella brine from the bag or water
3 medium eggs, beaten
olive oil, to grease

Preheat the oven to 200°C/180°C fan/400°F/gas mark 6 and line a baking tray with a silicone mat or baking parchment.

Use a large metal spoon to mix all the dry ingredients together in a large mixing bowl. Stir in the mozzarella, brine and then add the eggs. Alternatively, put the ingredients in a food processor and blitz until smooth. When you have a well combined thick dough (it will thicken as you mix), use your hands to gather it into a ball and remove it from the bowl.

Grease a work surface with a little oil. Divide the dough into 4 pieces and use your hands to roll them out into 4 evenly sized sausages about 24cm (9½in) long. Lay the baguettes on the baking tray at least 4cm (1½in) apart and flatten them to about 2.5cm (1in) thick.

Bake for 22 minutes or until lightly browned and firm to the touch. Remove from the oven and leave to cool on a rack before slicing and filling.

Per baguette: 7.1g net carbs, 10.4g fibre, 25.7g protein, 55.2g fat, 645kcal

Get ahead: The baguettes can be kept in the fridge for up to 4 days or covered and frozen for up to 3 months.

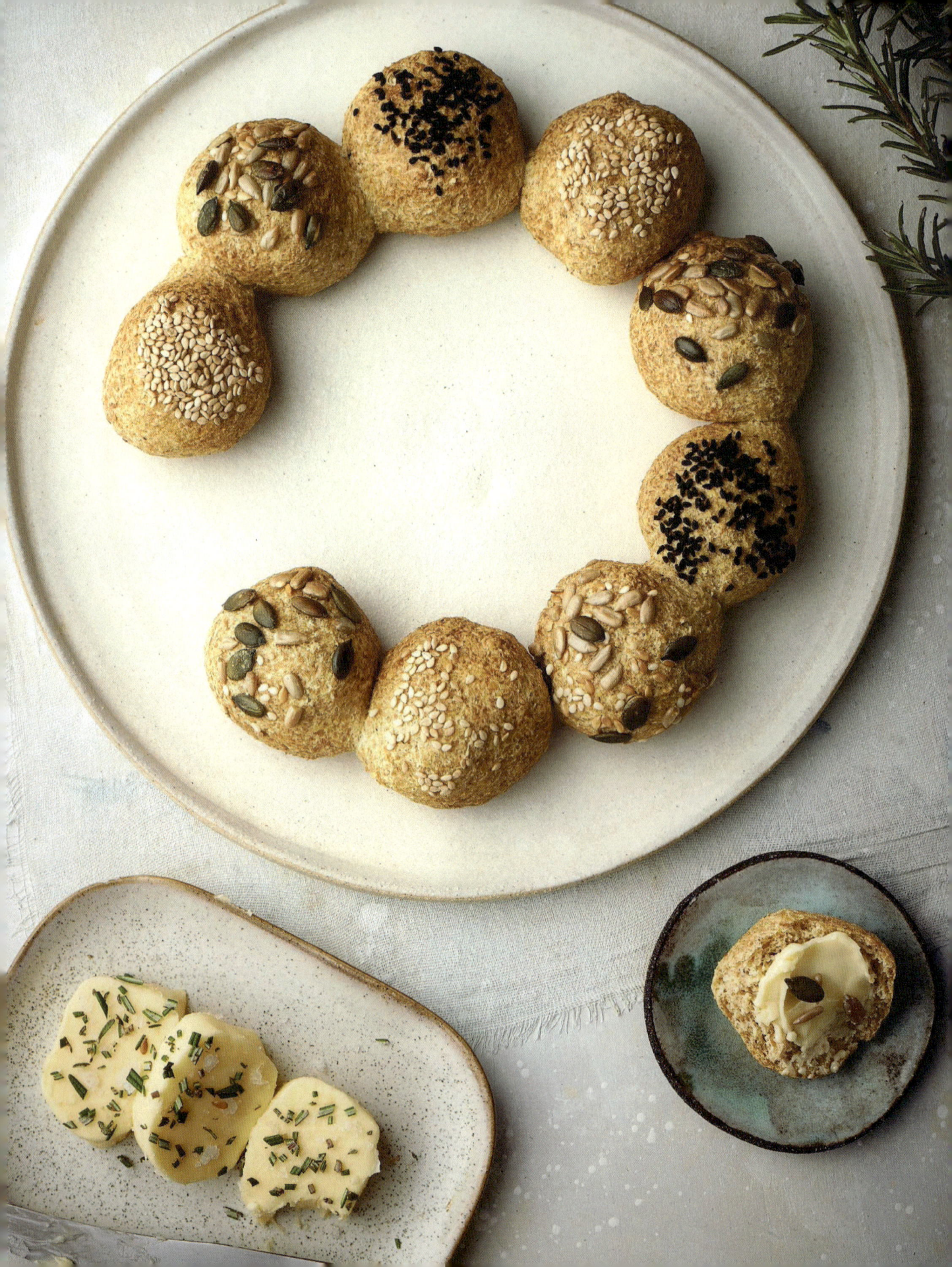

A Festive R... Rolls

These pretty little dinner roll... ...ve with soup or cheese. They are gluten and nut free and you can have fun with the flavours by altering the s...

Makes 10 mini rolls

20g (¾oz) coconut flour
10g (¼oz) psyllium husk
60g (2¼oz) golden flaxse...
1 teaspoon gluten-free ba...
½ teaspoon salt
1 medium egg
3 tablespoons seeds, such... ...nflower or sesame (optional)
olive oil, to grease

Preheat the oven to 220°C/200°C fan/425°F/gas mark 7 and grease a baking tray with a little oil.

Use a large metal spoon to mix all the dry ingredients together in a large mixing bowl. Crack the egg into the bowl and add 160ml (5½fl oz) cold water; stir through with a large spoon. When the dough is well combined, use your hands to bring it into a ball. It will thicken all the time as the water is absorbed. Now weigh the dough and divide it by the number of rolls you want to make. My dough weighs about 300g (10½oz) so I divide that by 10 so that I know each roll should be made from 30g (1oz) dough.

Put your chosen seeds into small saucers. Use lightly oiled hands to roll each piece into a ball and press the tops into the seeds. Put the rolls on to the baking tray spaced 1cm (1/2 in) apart.

Bake for 22-25 minutes or until lightly browned and firm to the touch. Remove from the oven and leave to cool on a rack before serving.

Per roll: 1.4g net carbs, 3.3 g fibre, 2.6g protein, 4.5g fat, 62kcal

Get ahead: The rolls will keep in the fridge for 3 days and can be frozen for up to 3 months.

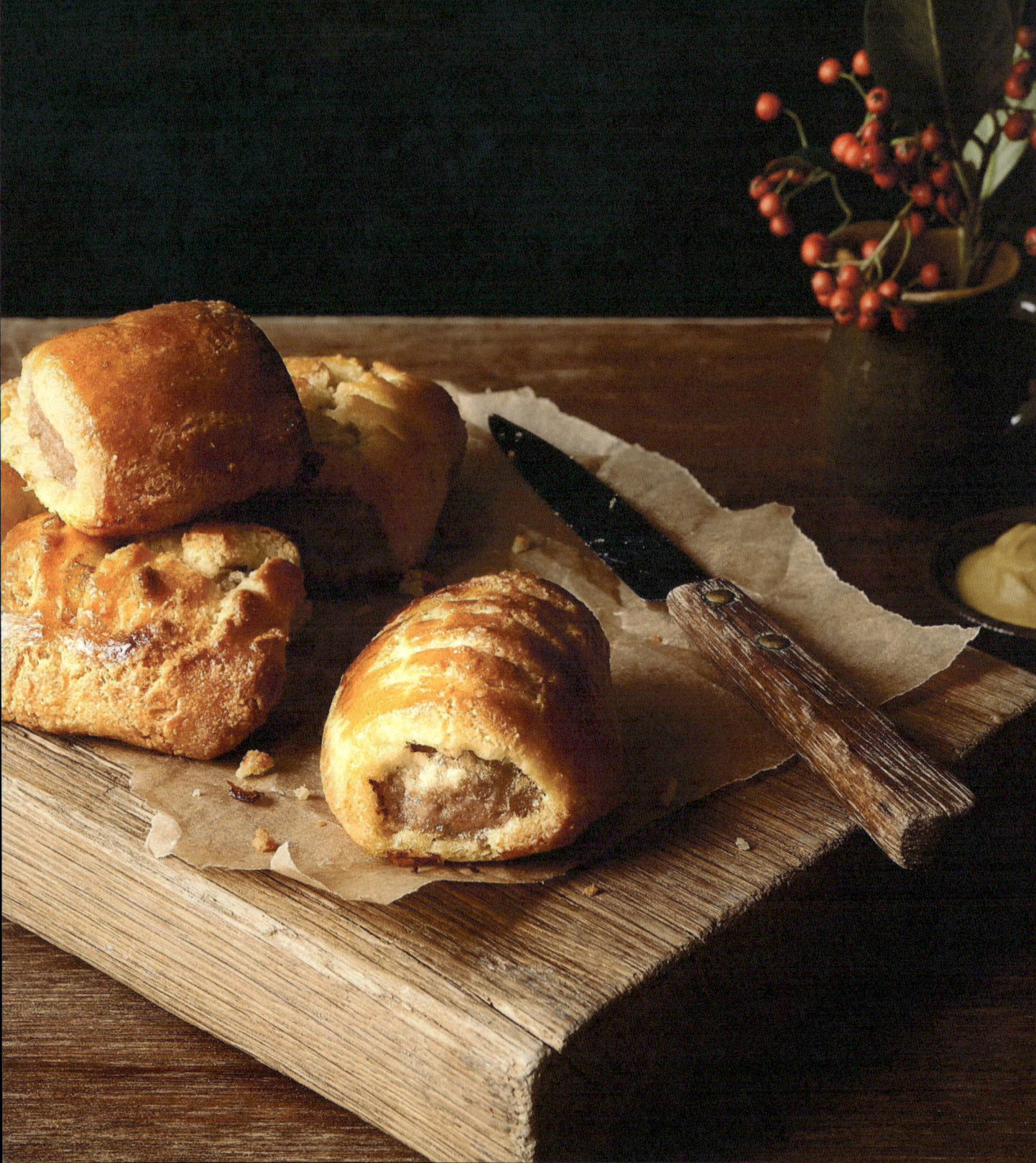

Sausage Rolls

Nutritionist Jenny Phillips asked me to create low-carb sausage rolls for her as her family has a tradition of eating them at Christmas. She used to peel off the pastry to avoid the gluten but I am happy to say this year she can now enjoy the whole sausage roll. Do seek out good-quality sausages with no or little added rusk (Italian sausages are good) and make sure you buy a gluten-free variety if you are gluten intolerant.

Makes 12 sausage rolls
6 high-meat content gluten-free sausages
1 egg yolk, beaten, to glaze

For the pastry
130g (4½oz) ground almonds
½ teaspoon xanthan gum
1 teaspoon baking powder
pinch of salt
30g (1oz) butter or lard, softened
1 egg

Preheat the oven to 200°C/180°C fan/400°F/gas mark 6 and cut two pieces of baking parchment the same size as a large baking tray.

Use a large metal spoon to mix the dry ingredients together for the pastry. Add the butter and egg and mix to form a smooth, well-blended dough. If your pastry is very dry, which can happen if your egg is small, add a tablespoon of water to help it bind together.

Use your hands to gather it into a ball and remove it from the bowl. Divide the pastry in half and gently roll each half into a sausage shape.

Place the dough sausages on one piece of baking parchment about 10cm (4in) apart. Lay the other piece of baking parchment on top and use a rolling pin to roll the sausages into two long, thin rectangles about 30 x 12cm (12 x 4½in) and 3mm (1/8in) thick. You can cut away misshapen pieces and add them in as necessary to make your rectangles. You shouldn't have any pastry left over.

Peel the skin from the sausages (or simply squeeze the meat out) and lay 3 along the centre of the rectangles. Obviously, some sausages are shorter or fatter than others, but you can squeeze or stretch the sausage meat out accordingly to fit the length. Use the parchment to roll up the pastry to cover the sausages. Trim the edges of the pastry as necessary. Cut each roll into 6 pieces. Use one piece of baking parchment to line the baking tray.

Lift the sausage rolls onto the prepared tray and brush with the egg yolk. Scatter over the sesame seeds, if using. Bake for 20 minutes until the pastry is golden brown. Remove from the oven and serve the sausage rolls warm or at room temperature. Once cooled they will keep in the fridge for up to 3 days in a container. They also freeze for up to 3 months.

Per roll: 1.4g net carbs, 1.3g fibre, 4.7g protein, 11.2g fat, 130kcal

Get ahead: The rolls will keep in the fridge for 3 days and can be frozen for up to 3 months.

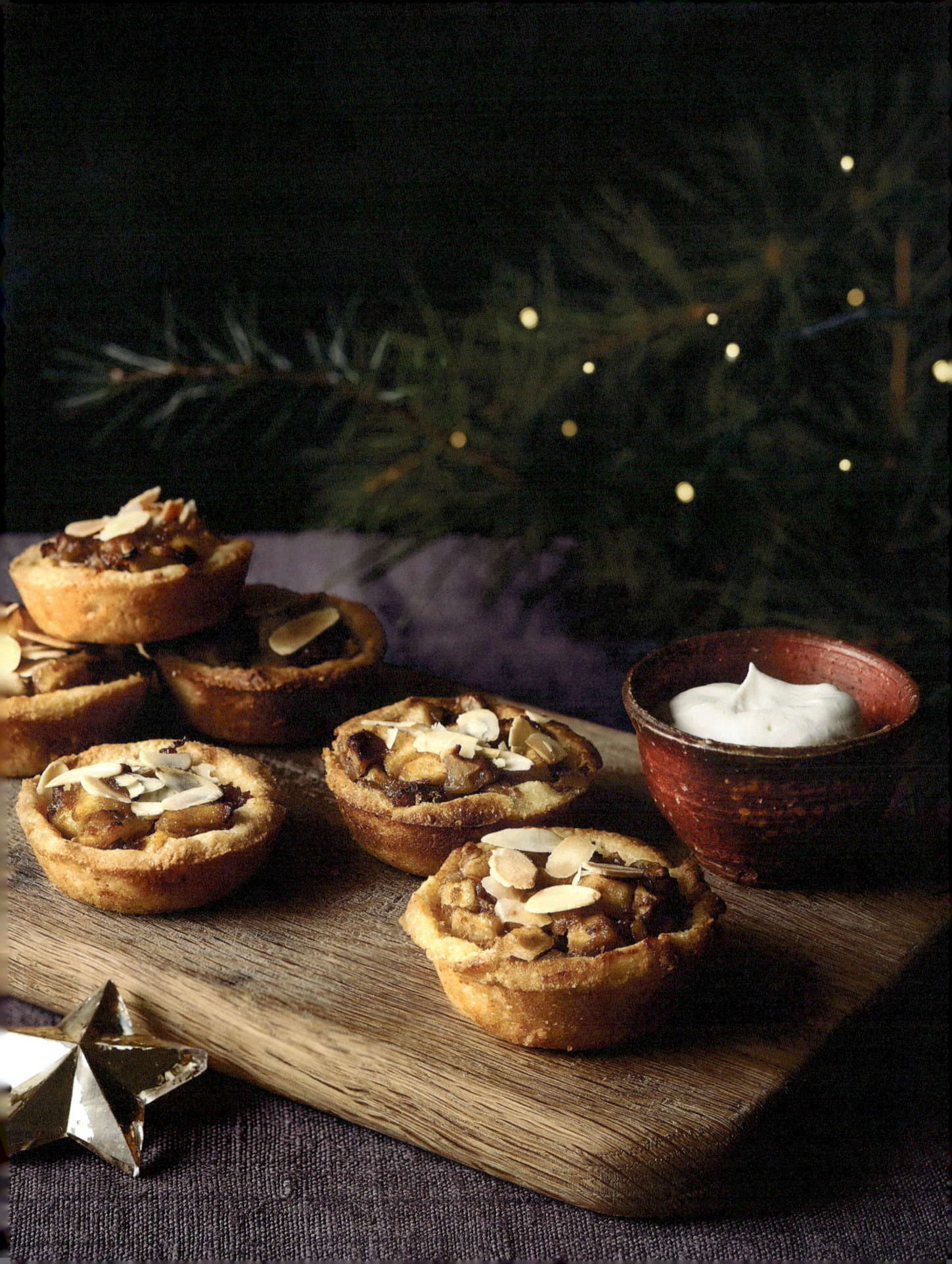

Chapter Four

Desserts & Sweet Treats

Our tastes have changed over the years and now we find many foods too sweet, but it is difficult not to use any sweetness at all when you are making desserts. We have gone from liking milk chocolate to loving 90% dark chocolate and never have sugar in tea and coffee any more. Desserts are a treat and not an everyday occurrence, so we don't feel bad indulging occasionally.

We use unsalted butter for our desserts and medium sized eggs. Instead of using a shop-bought spice blend such as Mixed Spice I have used cinnamon, cloves, nutmeg and ginger. I find the combination more controllable and flavour superior. Buy the best vanilla extract you can afford preferably without added sugar; I use abundantly as it gives a sweet flavour.

Some people are anti artificial sweeteners, others are against any form of sugar, including more natural forms such as honey. You have to make your choice; for more information on sweeteners see our website www.lowcarbtogether.com and in the introduction. In this chapter we have chosen to use honey, treacle or erythritol in small quantities to add sweetness.

You will see that we use ground almonds in baking instead of flour. The darker ground almonds are made from whole almonds whereas the paler versions are made from blanched almonds and sometimes called almond flour – these are useful when you want a very pale result such as in the [Coconut, Rum & Lime Trifle.](#)

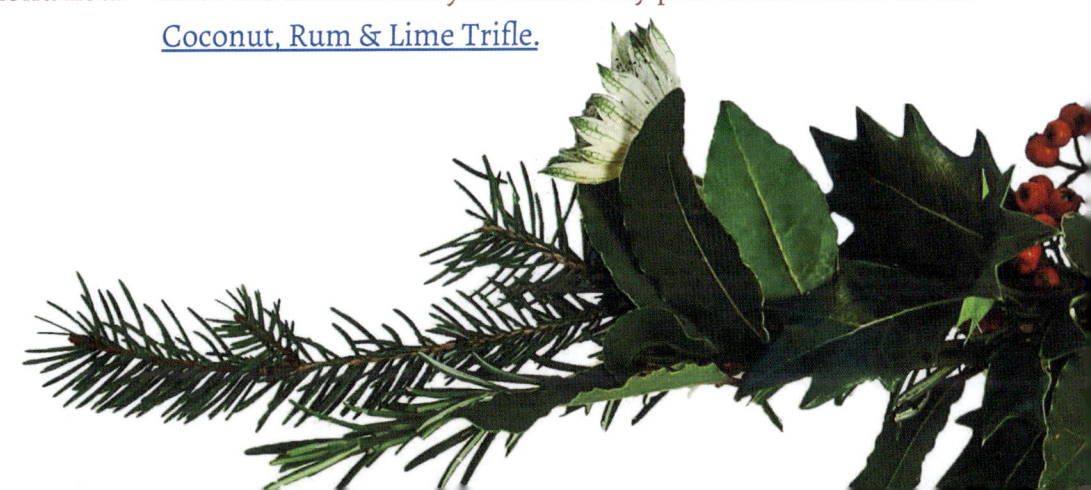

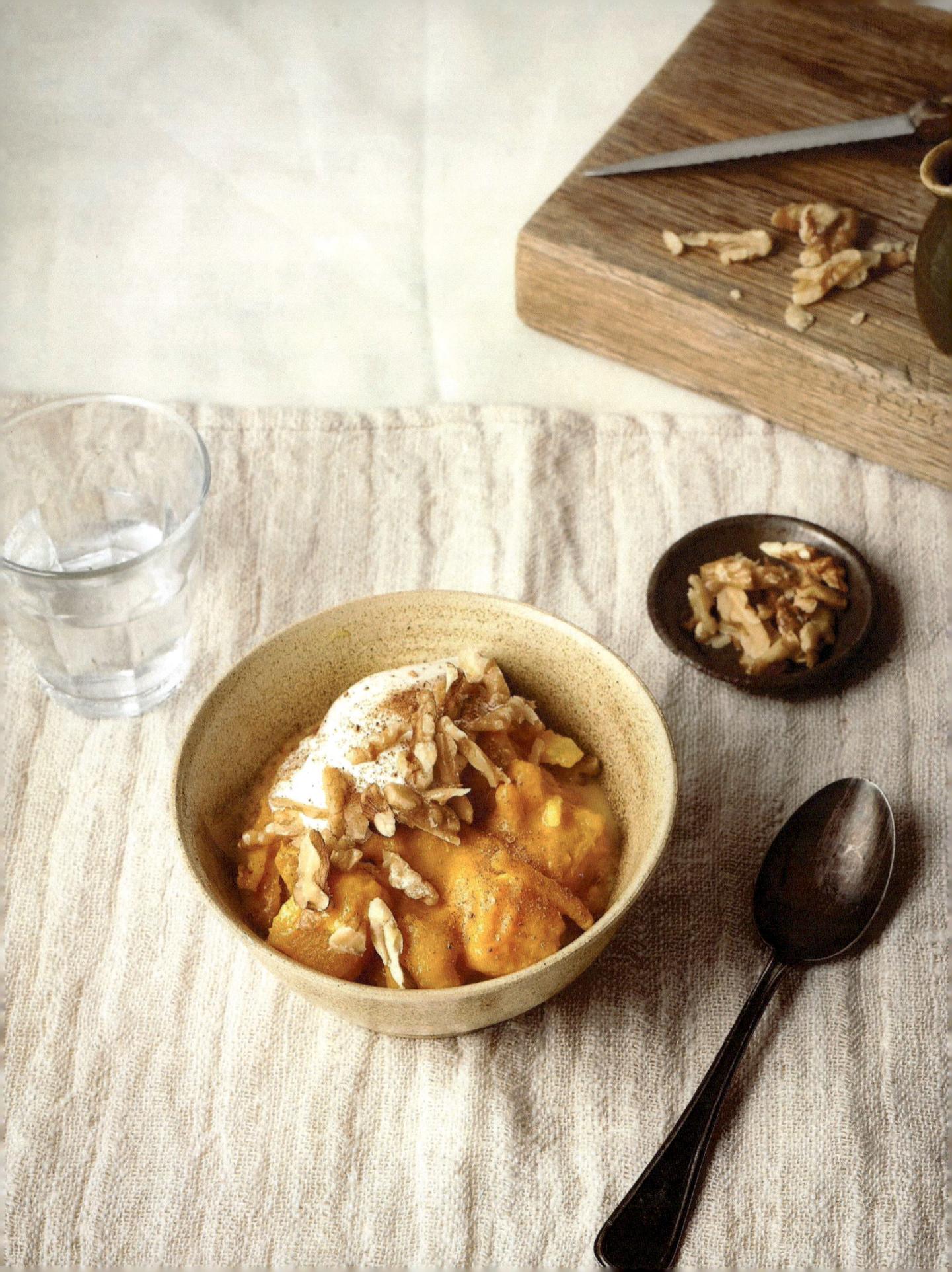

Pumpkin Porridge

Do try to find a cooking pumpkin such as a kabocha or crown prince for their firm and waxy flesh. The jack-o'-lantern orange pumpkins for carving don't have such a good texture to eat and can be watery. This recipe makes 4 small portions which we have from the fridge for breakfast. If we cook the pumpkin in coconut milk, we don't add any extra sweetness as it doesn't need it. The extra pumpkin keeps well in the fridge for up to a week; it's wonderful roasted or [mashed like the swede.](#)

Serves 4

600g (1lb 5oz) pumpkin
300ml (10fl oz) almond, cow's or coconut milk or water
4 cloves (optional)
1 cinnamon stick
50g (1¾oz) fresh ginger, peeled and julienned
1 tablespoon vanilla extract
2 teaspoons maple syrup or honey or 3 tablespoons erythritol (optional)
very small pinch of salt

Peel the pumpkin by cutting the skin away or peeling with a sharp potato peeler. Cut the flesh into 2cm (¾in) cubes. Put the cubes and the remaining ingredients into a saucepan and bring to the boil. Cover and reduce the heat to a gentle boil. Cook, shaking and stirring the pan frequently, for 10–15 minutes or until the pumpkin becomes soft and tender but not mushy. Different pumpkins will take less or more time to cook.

Serve warm or cold on its own or with full-fat Greek yogurt, walnuts and a dusting of cinnamon.

Per serving made with almond milk and including maple syrup: 9.8g net carbs, 1.8g fibre, 1.4g protein, 0.9g fat, 54kcal
Per serving made with coconut milk and excluding maple syrup: 8.6g net carbs, 1.7g fibre, 1.2g protein, 1.5g fat, 48kcal

Get ahead: Keep the porridge in the fridge for 3 days or freeze for up to 3 months.

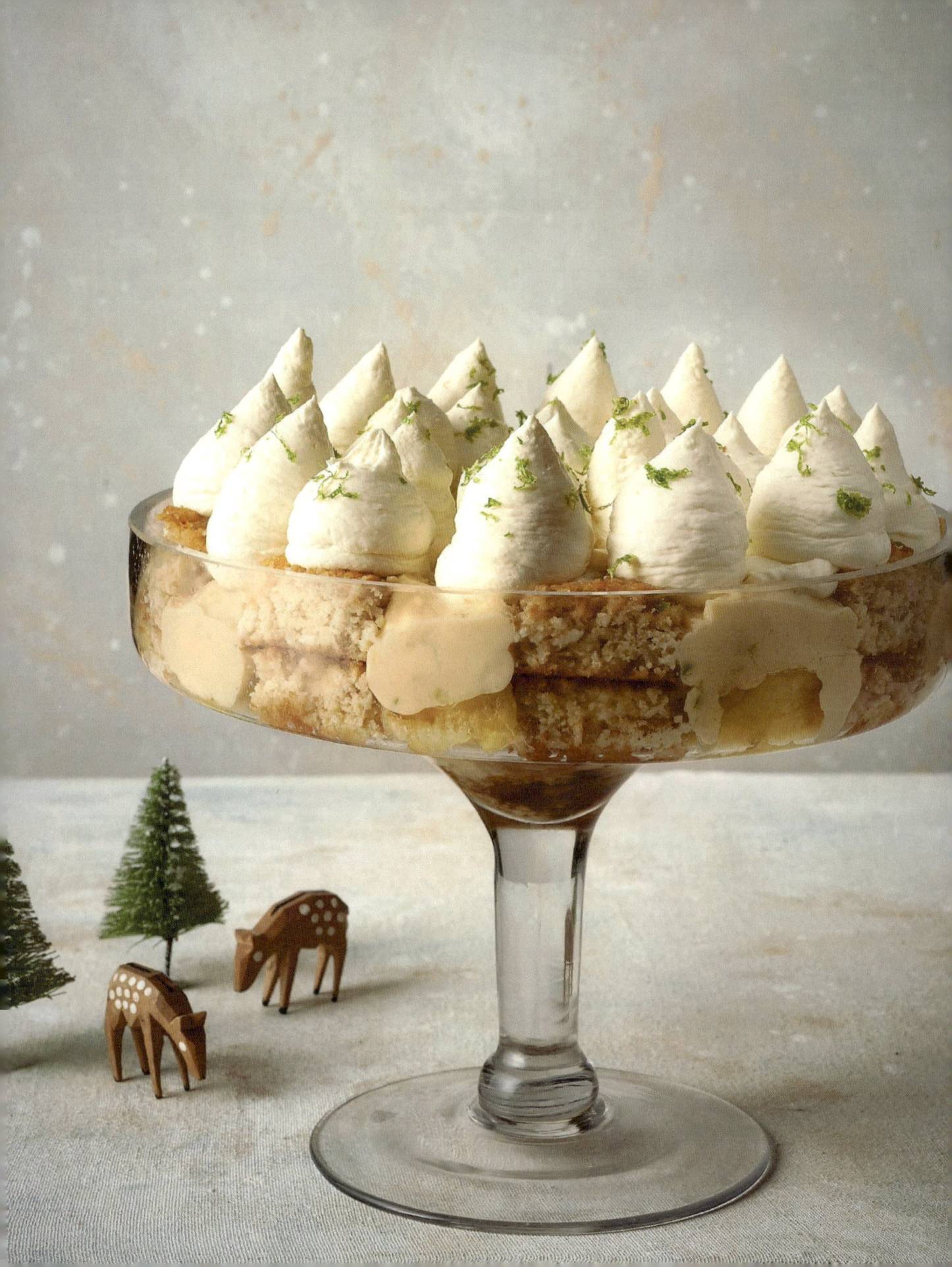

Coconut, Rum & Lime Trifle

Buttery coconut cake meets sweet pineapple and lime custard in a cloud of vanilla whipped cream in this impressive celebration trifle. The cake base works perfectly as a trifle sponge or is delicious on its own with a cup of tea. By using the natural sweetness of coconut, you can reduce any additional sweeteners to a minimum.

Serves 8

For the cake
100g (3 ½ fl oz) unsalted butter, melted, plus extra for greasing
50g (1 ¾ oz) ground almonds
50g (1 ¾ oz) desiccated coconut
15g (½ oz) coconut flour
1 teaspoon gluten-free baking powder
100ml (3 ½ fl oz) double cream
2 teaspoons vanilla extract
2 teaspoons honey or tablespoons erythritol
1 egg yolk
2 medium egg whites

For the lime custard
1 quantity of Vanilla Custard (without the bay leaves)
finely grated zest of 2 limes

For the trifle
150g (5 ½ oz) pineapple chunks
7 tablespoons dark rum
250ml (9fl oz) whipped cream
1 teaspoon vanilla extract
juice of 2 limes, plus zest of 1

Preheat the oven to 190° C/170 ° C fan/375° F/gas mark 5, grease a 20cm (8in) tin generously with butter and cut a circle of baking parchment to fit the base.

To make the cake, mix the dry ingredients together in a bowl with a large metal spoon. Now add the cream, butter, vanilla, sweetener and egg yolk and stir through.

Beat the egg whites with an electric whisk until they form stiff peaks. Use the mixer to whisk a little of the egg whites into the cake batter to loosen it. Then switch to a large metal spoon and fold the remaining egg whites in. Be gentle and don't overmix it.

Spoon the batter into the prepared tin and bake for 20 minutes or until golden brown and a skewer inserted into the centre comes out clean. Remove from the oven and leave to cool in the tin for 15 minutes. Run a dinner knife around the edge to loosen the cake before carefully turning it out on to a wire rack to cool to room temperature.

Meanwhile, make the custard and when it is cooked stir in the lime zest. When the cake has cooled, cut it into smaller shapes and arrange in your trifle dish with the pineapple. Mix the rum with 2 tablespoons of water and pour over the sponge, followed by the custard and spread it out to the edges.

Whip the cream with the vanilla and lime juice until soft peaks form and spoon over the trifle or use a piping bag to pipe it over. Scatter over the lime zest. Put the trifle into the fridge for a few hours for the cream to firm up and for the rum to soak into the sponge.

Per serving: 10g net carbs, 2.3g fibre, 4.3g protein, 28.5g fat, 347kcal
Per serving without honey: 6.4g net carbs, 2.3g fibre, 4.3g protein, 28.5.6g fat, 334kcal
Get ahead: To get ahead of time you can make and freeze the sponge in advance. The trifle can be assembled minus the cream the day before and kept in the fridge.

Vanilla Custard

This is delicious over the Spiced Christmas Pudding if you aren't making the Marmalade. It is also used in the Coconut, Rum & Lime Trifle. To reduce the carb count by 3g, use almond milk as it doesn't contain the milk sugar lactose. If you can't eat egg, you can use ready-made sugar-free custard powder. A recent discovery is Bay Custard, it has a gentle herbal spice, perfect for Christmas.

Serves 6

1 tablespoon honey or 3 tablespoons erythritol
500ml (18fl oz) unsweetened almond or cow's milk
4 egg yolks
2 teaspoons vanilla extract
15g (½oz) cornflour
4 small bay leaves, optional

Whisk the ingredients together in a saucepan (off the heat) until completely smooth. Add the bay leaves if you are making Bay Custard. Put the saucepan over a gentle heat and bring to the boil, whisking continuously. Reduce the heat to medium and continue to cook until smooth and thickened. Remove from the heat. Leave the bay leaves in the custard until the flavour is strong enough. If not using straight away, cover the surface with dampened baking parchment to stop it forming a skin.

Per serving with almond milk and honey: 6.1g net carbs, 0.2g fibre, 2g protein, 3.4g fat, 63kcal
Per serving with almond milk and no honey: 3.2g net carbs, 0.2g fibre, 2g protein, 3.4g fat, 52kcal

Get ahead: The custard can be made in advance and, after cooling to room temperature, can be stored in the fridge for up to 2 days.

Christmas Cookies

These simple cookies have all the flavour of Christmas from the mixed spice and ginger. They are good as a small sweet end to a meal instead of a pudding or try them with the [Eggnog.](#)

Makes 10 cookies approx. 5cm (2in)

50g (1¾oz) walnuts
1 medium carrot (approx. 70g/2½oz) carrot, coarsely grated
50g (1¾oz) unsalted butter
100g (3½oz) ground almonds
1 medium egg
2 teaspoons honey or 2 tablespoons erythritol
1 teaspoon vanilla extract
½ teaspoon gluten-free baking powder
1 heaped teaspoon ground ginger
1 heaped teaspoon mixed spice

Preheat the oven to 190°C/170°C fan/375°F/gas mark 5. Put the walnuts on a tray and toast them in the oven for 4 minutes. Remove from the oven and leave to cool.

Line a baking tray with baking parchment or a silicone mat.

Roughly chop the walnuts into a bowl with a cook's knife and stir in the remaining ingredients to form a dough. Take walnut-sized balls of dough and roll them into balls. Lay them on the prepared tray and flatten into cookies about 5cm (2in) in diameter. Bake for 10–12 minutes or until lightly browned.

Remove from the oven and leave to cool on the tray. Serve straight away or leave to cool and keep in an airtight container for up to 4 days. If the cookies become soft, simply put them into a hot oven for a few minutes to dry out.

Per cookie: 1.6g net carbs, 0.3g fibre, 1.4g protein, 7.8g fat, 81kcal
Per cookie without honey: 0.5g net carbs, 0.3g fibre, 1.4g protein, 7.8g fat, 76kcal

Get ahead: These can be prepared and cooked in advance. Once cooled, they can be frozen and kept for up to 3 months. Defrost to room temperature and have them as they are or briefly re-heat in the oven if soft.

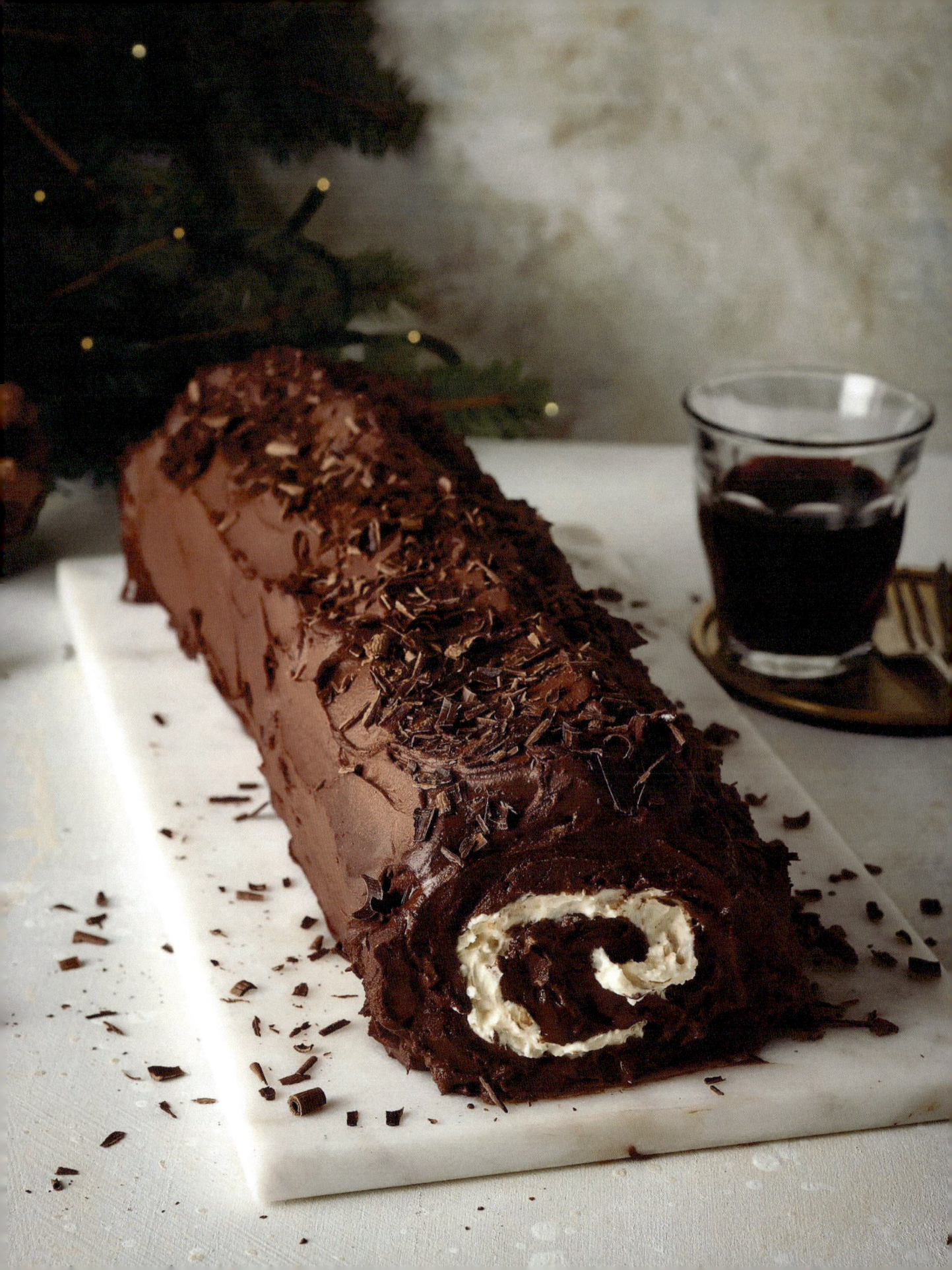

Chocolate Yule Log

Yule logs date back to the Iron Age when people would celebrate the end of the longest days and welcome in the spring. They would burn logs decorated with holly, pine cones or ivy or even wine and salt. Eventually, as hearths became obsolete in most homes, wooden logs were replaced with cakes in a log shape. With the help of patisserie chef Stefano Borella, we have made a rich and indulgent Yule Log that takes its sweetness from the chocolate.

Serves 12

For the sponge
4 medium eggs
35g (1¼oz) cocoa powder
75g (2½oz) ground almonds
2 teaspoon honey or 2 tablespoons erythritol
3 tablespoons almond or cow's milk
1 heaped teaspoon gluten-free baking powder
2 teaspoons vanilla extract

For the filling
150ml (5fl oz) whipping cream
2 teaspoons vanilla extract
1 teaspoon honey or 1 tablespoon erythritol
75g fresh or frozen raspberries, defrosted

For the chocolate coating
200ml (7fl oz) whipping cream
2 teaspoons vanilla extract
135g (4¾oz) dark chocolate
(85% cocoa solids), plus extra for the shavings

Preheat the oven to 200°C/180°C fan/400°F/gas mark 6. You will need a Swiss roll tin or shallow baking tray about 33 x 23cm (13 x 9in). You can form this shape from a larger tin by using a folded length of foil to block off part of the tin to make the right shape if necessary. Line the tin with baking parchment.

To make the sponge, separate the eggs and put the yolks in one mixing bowl and the whites in another. Sift the cocoa powder into the bowl with the yolks and add the ground almonds, sweetener, milk, baking powder and vanilla. Mix together thoroughly with a metal spoon.

Whisk the egg whites with an electric whisk until stiff peaks form. Add 2 tablespoons of the whisked egg whites to the almond mixture and whisk it in with the electric whisk. Then switch to a large metal spoon to gently fold in the remaining egg whites. Spoon on to the prepared baking tray and spread out with a palette knife until 5m (¼in) thick.

Bake for 8 minutes or until the sponge is just firm to the touch. Remove from the oven and invert the tin on to a clean tea towel. Shunt the sponge to one long edge and roll the sponge up into a tight spiral with the cloth. Leave to cool, covered in the cloth, with the edge down so that it sets into this shape.

To make the chocolate shavings, use a vegetable peeler to scrape chocolate shavings (while it is still in a bar) into a bowl set on some scales. You will need 10g (¼oz). Put the bowl in the fridge to keep the shavings cool.

Break the remaining chocolate into small pieces and put into a mixing bowl. Warm the cream and vanilla in a small saucepan over a medium heat. When warm, remove the pan from the heat and pour over the chocolate. Use a whisk to blend the chocolate into the warm cream. Set aside to cool. After 10 minutes you can put it into the fridge to speed up the cooling.

To make the filling, whisk the cream, vanilla and sweetener together in a bowl with a whisk until firm.

When the sponge is cool to the touch, remove the cloth and carefully unfurl the sponge. Spread the filling evenly over the surface using a palette knife, leaving a 2cm (¾in) border around the edges. Scatter over the raspberries, breaking them up a little with your fingers if they are large.

Use the parchment to roll up the sponge lengthways around the cream to create a spiral. It should overlap slightly to seal in the cream. Arrange the roulade on a serving platter with the seam underneath.

Spoon the chocolate coating over the log and use a palette knife to create the texture of bark. Scatter over the chocolate shavings. Put into the fridge to chill for a minimum of 1 hour and up to a day before serving. Just before serving add your decoration as you wish.

Per serving with honey: 8.3g net carbs, 2.1g fibre, 5.6g protein, 19.5g fat, 231kcal
Per serving with no honey: 6.8g net carbs, 2.1g fibre, 5.6 protein, 19.5g fat, 225kcal

Get ahead: The Yule Log can be made a day before you need it. Leftovers keep well in the fridge for 3 days.

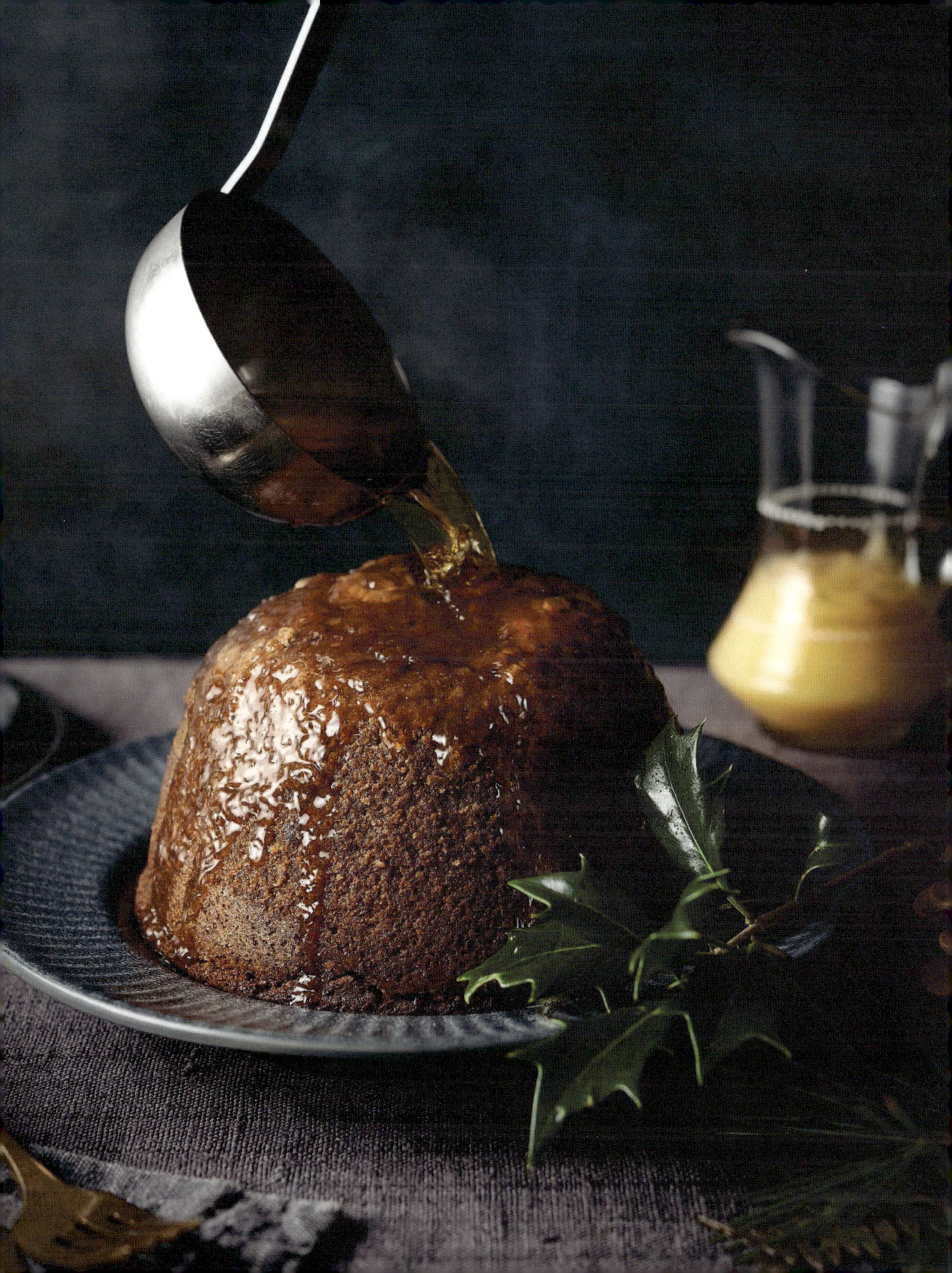

Spiced Christmas Pudding with Hot Marmalade Sauce

The typical Christmas pudding has around 57g (2oz) carbs per portion, so it is not great for your blood sugar levels. Traditionally a pudding is full of dried fruits, sugar and breadcrumbs, probably one of the most carb-heavy desserts around. However, I like a challenge and I am really proud of this one. We have made a gorgeous alternative that feels every bit as indulgent with just a fraction of the carbs.

We have used sticky black treacle to sweeten the pudding; it is a form of sugar, but we think the colour and flavour it adds is worth the carbs and it is used in minimal quantities. We have made a bright, zesty orange sauce from the [Marmalade](#) recipe which is gorgeous with the pudding with clouds of whipped cream, but you could simply serve this with pouring cream or the [Vanilla and Bay Custard](#). Use the spare orange juice for the [Wonky Madonna](#) cocktail.

Serves 8

For the sponge pudding

50g (2 oz) (30g (1 1/8 oz) raisins
2 tablespoons rum (optional)
2 tablespoons brandy (optional)
50g whole blanched almonds
100 (3 ½oz) unsalted butter, softened, plus extra to grease
2 tablespoons black treacle or honey or 6 tablespoons erythritol
1 apple, cored and cut into 1cm (3/8")
75g (2½oz) walnuts

2 medium eggs
100g (5oz) ground almonds
2 teaspoons vanilla extract
zest and juice of 1 orange
zest of 1 lemon
1 heaped tablespoon ground ginger
½ teaspoon ground nutmeg
½ teaspoon ground cloves
2 teaspoons cinnamon
2 teaspoons gluten-free baking powder

For the marmalade sauce

200ml (7fl oz) [marmalade](#)
4 tablespoons brandy or whisky to flame the pudding (optional)

Soak the raisins in the brandy and rum. Soak the almonds in hot water.

Preheat the oven to 190°C/170°C fan/375°F/gas mark 5. Generously grease a 1 litre (35 fl oz) pudding basin or ovenproof bowl (we have used a pyrex measuring jug before) with butter and put a disc of baking parchment at the bottom. Prepare a lid for the pudding basin by cutting a circle of baking parchment big enough to cover the basin with at least 2.5cm (1") overlap. Cut a circle of foil the same size. Butter the baking parchment on one side.

Put the remaining ingredients for the sponge pudding into a mixing bowl. Drain the almonds and add them to the bowl with the raisins and alcohol. Spoon the mixture into the pudding basin. There should be around a two-finger width gap between the top of the pudding and the brim of the basin.

Lay the circle of parchment buttered side down over the top of the pudding followed by the foil. Fold it down and tie it around the top with string. Put the pudding into a deep ovenproof dish and fill it with cold water to come up 5cm (2 in) around the sides of the basin. Bake for 2 hours or until the sponge is feels springy to the touch. Remove the pudding from the oven and leave it in a warm place until you are ready to serve for up to an hour.

To make the marmalade sauce, purée the marmalade with a stick blender, adding a little water as necessary to dilute it to a runny consistency. When you are ready to serve, heat it in a small pan or in the microwave briefly.

Lift the pudding basin out of the water. Run a knife around the edge of the basin and invert it on to a warm plate. Peel off the circle of parchment. Serve with the hot marmalade sauce in a jug on the side. To flame the pudding, warm the brandy in a small saucepan and leave a ladle in the pan to warm. Dim the lights and make sure you have everyone gathered and ready. Pour the brandy into the ladle and set it alight at arm's length. Pour over the pudding and serve straight away.

Per serving of pudding: 16.2g net carbs, 3.7g fibre, 7.4g protein, 27.6g fat, 362kcal
Per serving of pudding without the treacle and honey: 12.8g net carbs, 3.7g fibre, 7.3g protein, 27.6g fat, 349kcal
Get ahead: The pudding mix can be made a day in advance and kept in the fridge. The Marmalade Sauce can be made and kept in the fridge for up to a week.

Marmalade

Giancarlo and I love marmalade, so we have created this sugar-free version. It is lovely as it is, full of colour, zest and flavour. It makes a super gift for friends at Christmas but do tell them to keep it in the fridge as there is no sugar to preserve it. We love it with cream cheese on one of the [Festive Rolls](#) for breakfast. We have also used it puréed to create a bright orange pouring sauce for the [Spiced Christmas Pudding](#) and we also love it like this poured over a portion of chilled ricotta cheese.

Makes approx. 800ml (28fl oz)/3 small jars, serves 20

3 medium oranges
1 apple

Remove the hard-green part from the tops of the oranges and roughly chop them, peel, pith and all. Cut the apple into quarters and remove the core. Finely chop the fruit by hand or in a food processor into about 1cm (½in) pieces.

Put the fruit in a medium saucepan with 3 litres (5¼ pints) of water and bring to the boi Reduce the heat so the marmalade bubbles gently and cook for about 2 hours or until the skin softens easily when squashed against the side of the pan with a spoon, stirring occasionally. If it starts to dry out, add a little more water. By the end of cooking the marmalade should be like a soft-set jam. Remove from the heat and taste the marmalade. You may decide it is fine as it is but you can also add your chosen sweetener to taste.

Per serving with no sweetener: 3.5g net carbs; 0,7g fibre, 0g protein, 0g fat, 18kcal
Get ahead: The marmalade keeps in the fridge for up to 2 weeks.

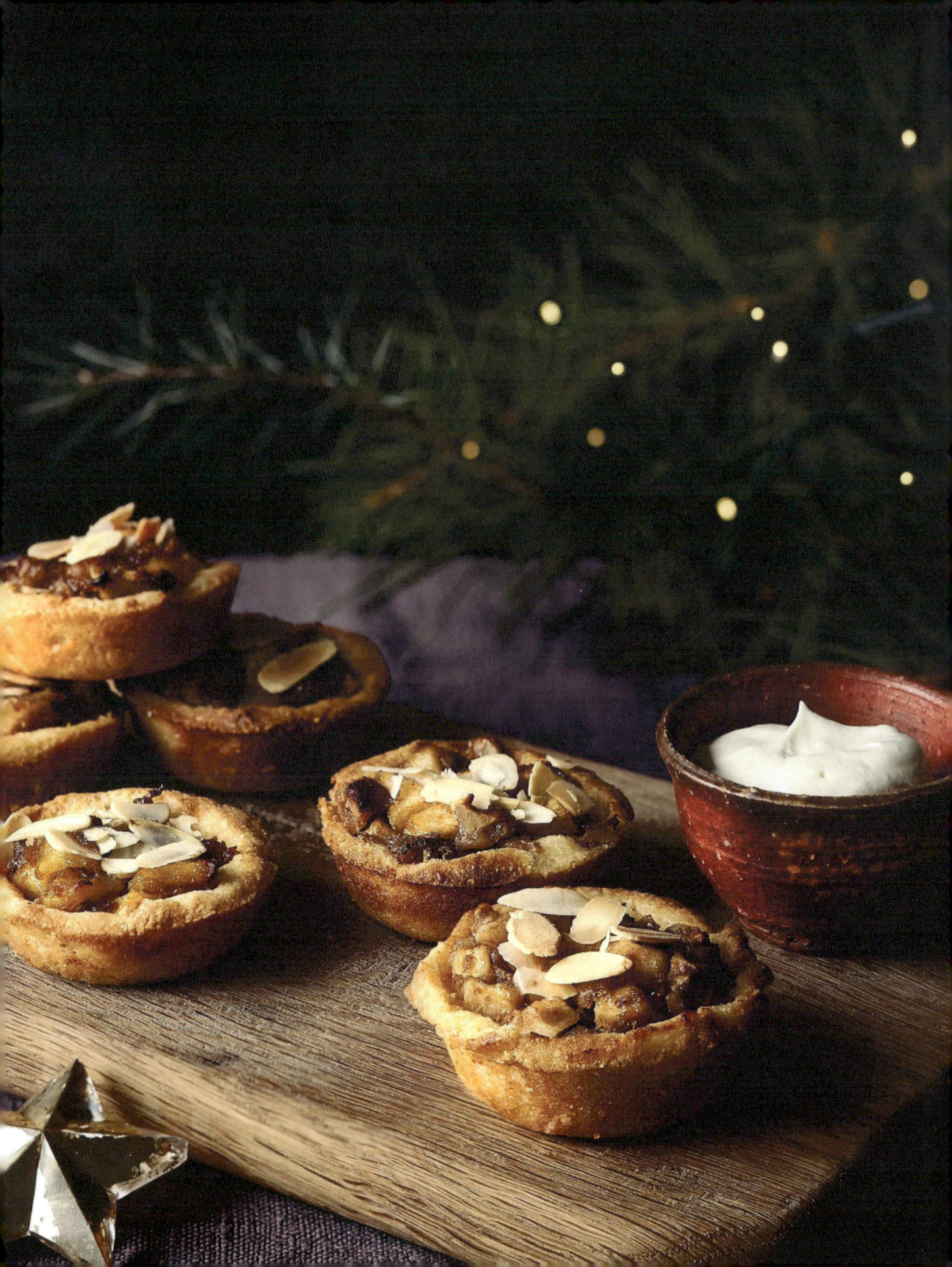

Mince Pies

Carol singing, glühwein and mince pies are still on the menu even if you are low-carb. Don't be surprised by the addition of mozzarella in the pastry – it is simply there to work as a binder and give strength to the pastry without adding any flavour. In a shop-bought mince pie you can expect to have 35 to 39g carbs but ours have only 10g. We have given a choice of sweeteners; black treacle gives a dark colour to the mincemeat and also adds a wonderful caramel flavour, while erythritol will add sweetness without sugar and calories. The choice is yours! We usually avoid raisins due to their high-sugar count but after many attempts, we decided it is the dried fruit that gives the familiar flavour to a mince pie. It is just not the same without them.

Makes 16

For the filling

2 apples, peeled and cut into 5mm (¼in) dice
50g (2oz) walnuts
60g (2 ¼ oz) raisins
2 tablespoon black treacle or 4 tablespoons erythritol
2 tablespoons honey or 4 tablespoons erythritol
2 tablespoons brandy or rum
4 teaspoons ginger powder
2 teaspoons cinnamon
½ teaspoon ground cloves
zest and juice of 2 oranges
15g flaked almonds

For the pastry

150g (5 ½ oz) ground almonds
125g (4 ½ oz) cow's milk mozzarella, coarsely grated
1 medium egg
50g (1 ¾ oz) unsalted butter
1 teaspoon honey or 1 tablespoon erythritol
1 teaspoon vanilla extract

Preheat the oven to 190°C/170°C fan/375°F/gas mark 5. Grease shallow pie tins with butter.

To make the pastry, mix all the ingredients together in a food processor or by hand in a mixing bowl. Divide the pastry into 16 even-sized balls and push them into the pie tin so that the pastry is about 5mm (¼in) thick.

Put the ingredients for the filling into a saucepan and bring the mixture to the boil, stirring frequently. Reduce the heat to medium and cook for 10 minutes until almost all of the orange juice has disappeared and the mixture has thickened. Spoon the filling into the pastry moulds, top with the flaked almonds and cook for 17 to 20 minutes or until golden brown and firm to the touch. Serve warm or at room temperature.

Per pie: 10g net carbs, 1.8g fibre, 4.7g protein, 12g fat, 175kcal
Per pie without honey and treacle: 6.6g net carbs, 1.8g fibre, 4.7g protein, 12g fat, 158kcal

Get ahead: The pies can be made in advance and frozen or stored at room temperature for up to 3 days in an airtight container.

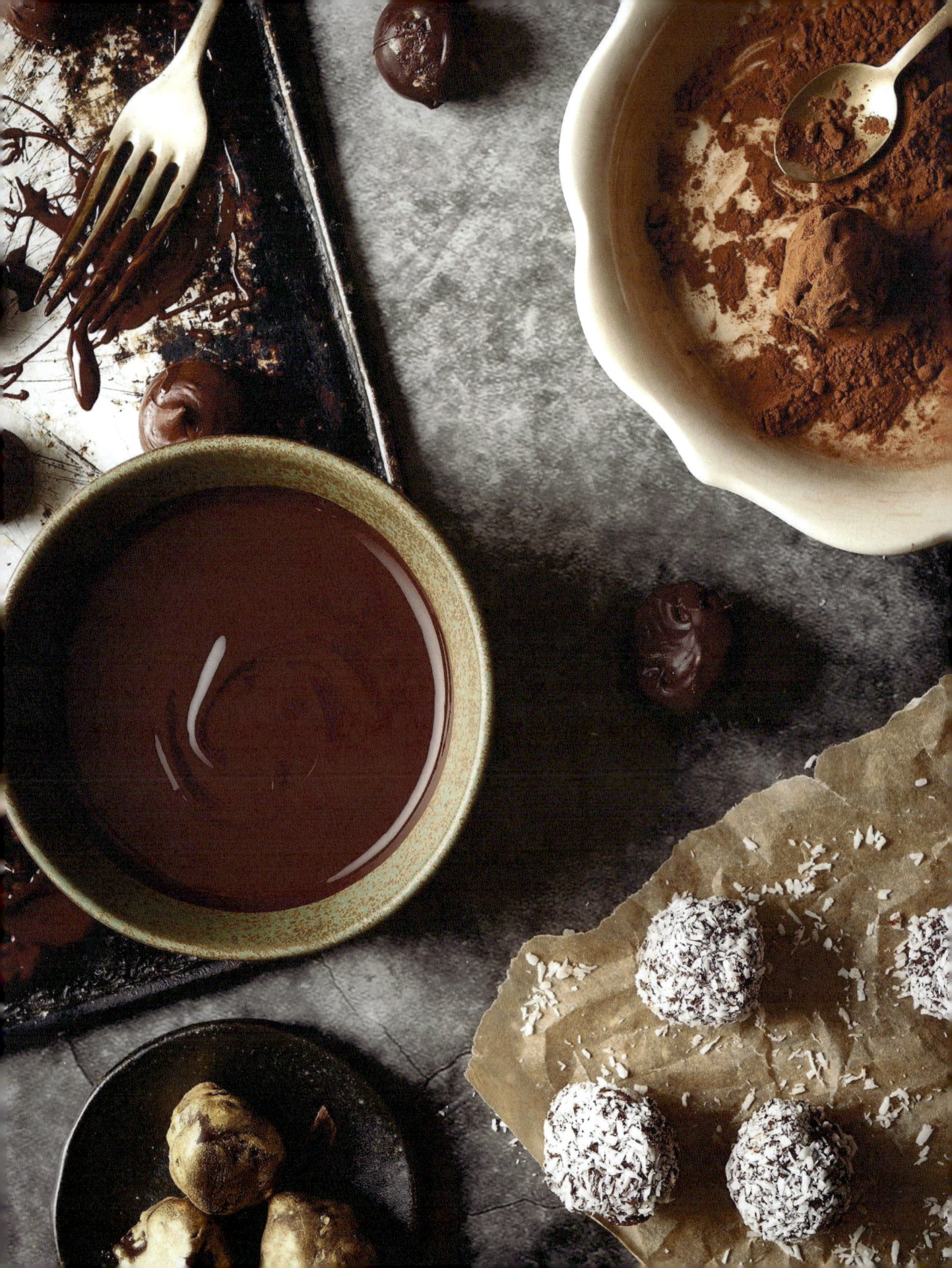

Chocolate Truffles

Stefano Borella, patisserie chef and head teacher at our cookery school suggests the following way to get the best out of your chocolate work.

There are types of bakers' chocolate available with added lecithin that make this process easier, but the flavour is not as good. All good-quality chocolate is tempered to make it into a bar or block. To work with chocolate, you need to melt it, which un-tempers it. Therefore, it needs to be re-tempered to crystallise the fats.

Tempering Chocolate

Make sure the bowl you use is completely dry and scrupulously clean as the chocolate must not come into contact with water. Heat the chocolate to roughly 40–45°C (100–115°F) in the microwave or over a bain-marie, making sure you don't burn it. If you don't have a thermometer, take it out a little before it is completely melted and stir to dissolve the remaining lumps.

Overheating it will result in grainy chocolate. If you are using a bain-marie, as soon as the water comes to the boil, take it off the heat, then put the bowl containing the chocolate on top. Ensure that no steam comes up around the edges of the bowl. Cool it down, stirring frequently, and leave it to cool to 28–30°C (82–86°F). It will change consistency slightly and start to thicken.

To check whether it is tempered, brush a little chocolate on to a piece of baking parchment. It should set within 5 minutes at room temperature and be glossy and even. If you look carefully at the surface, there should be no streaks of fat. When it has reached the tempering stage, use it straight away or reheat it momentarily to 31–32°C (88–90°F) to make it easier to work with .(Experienced pastry chefs test to see if it is ready by dabbing a little on their lower lip.) You can reheat chocolate up to four or five times; after that, it will deteriorate but it can still be used for a sauce or ganache.

How to make chocolate truffles

Makes about 35 truffles

125ml (4fl oz) whipping or pouring cream
1 teaspoon vanilla extract
125g (4½oz) dark chocolate (85% cocoa solids), roughly chopped
25g (1oz) unsalted butter, cubed and at room temperature

For the coating

175g (6oz) dark chocolate (85% cocoa solids)
50g (1¾oz) desiccated coconut
25g (1oz) cocoa powder
edible gold lustre powder

Put the cream and vanilla extract in a saucepan and bring to the boil. This can also be done rapidly in a microwave. Remove from the heat and leave to cool until it reaches 65–70°C (149–158°F).

Melt the chocolate in a bowl over a bain-marie to about 45°C (113°F) and remove the bowl from the heat. Gradually add the cooled cream and the butter to the chocolate, mixing constantly with a spatula to form a glossy emulsion. This is your ganache. Leave it to cool for about 1 hour to firm up.

Spoon the ganache into a piping bag and pipe about 35 mounds on to a piece of baking parchment on a tray. (If you don't have a piping bag, use 2 teaspoons to form mounds instead.) They should be just bigger than a marble. Put the tray into the fridge to set firm for 1 hour.

Now t[emper the chocolate](#) to make the coating. While the chocolate is still warm and runny, use 2 forks to pick up the mounds of ganache and drop them one by one into the bowl. Toss them around gently with the forks and transfer them back on to the baking parchment to set firm for a few minutes if you are leaving them plain or dust with edible gold powder. If you wish to coat them in coconut or cocoa powder, drop them from the forks into a bowl of your chosen coating. Roll them around in the coating and set back on to the baking parchment. The chocolates are now ready to eat.

Per serving without outer coating: 1.4g net carbs, 0.6g fibre, 0.6g protein, 3.6g fat, 40kcal

Get ahead: Prepare the truffles and keep them in a cool place for up to 5 days.

Chapter 5

Cocktails & Drinks

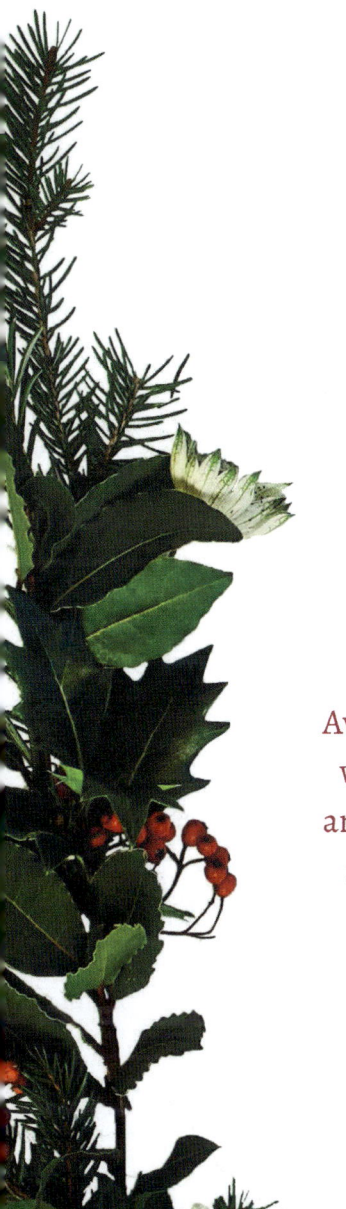

Drinks can easily contain hidden sugars so be careful what you consume over the festive period or try the cocktails in this chapter. Avoid sugary mixers and beer and stick to champagne, dry white or red wine with plenty of glasses of water between. Not all sparkling wines are dry, so do check the label. Have a [Smoky Mary](#), particularly if you've made the chilli vodka for the [Savoy Pasta with Hot-smoked Salmon, Cream & Chilli Vodka.](#)

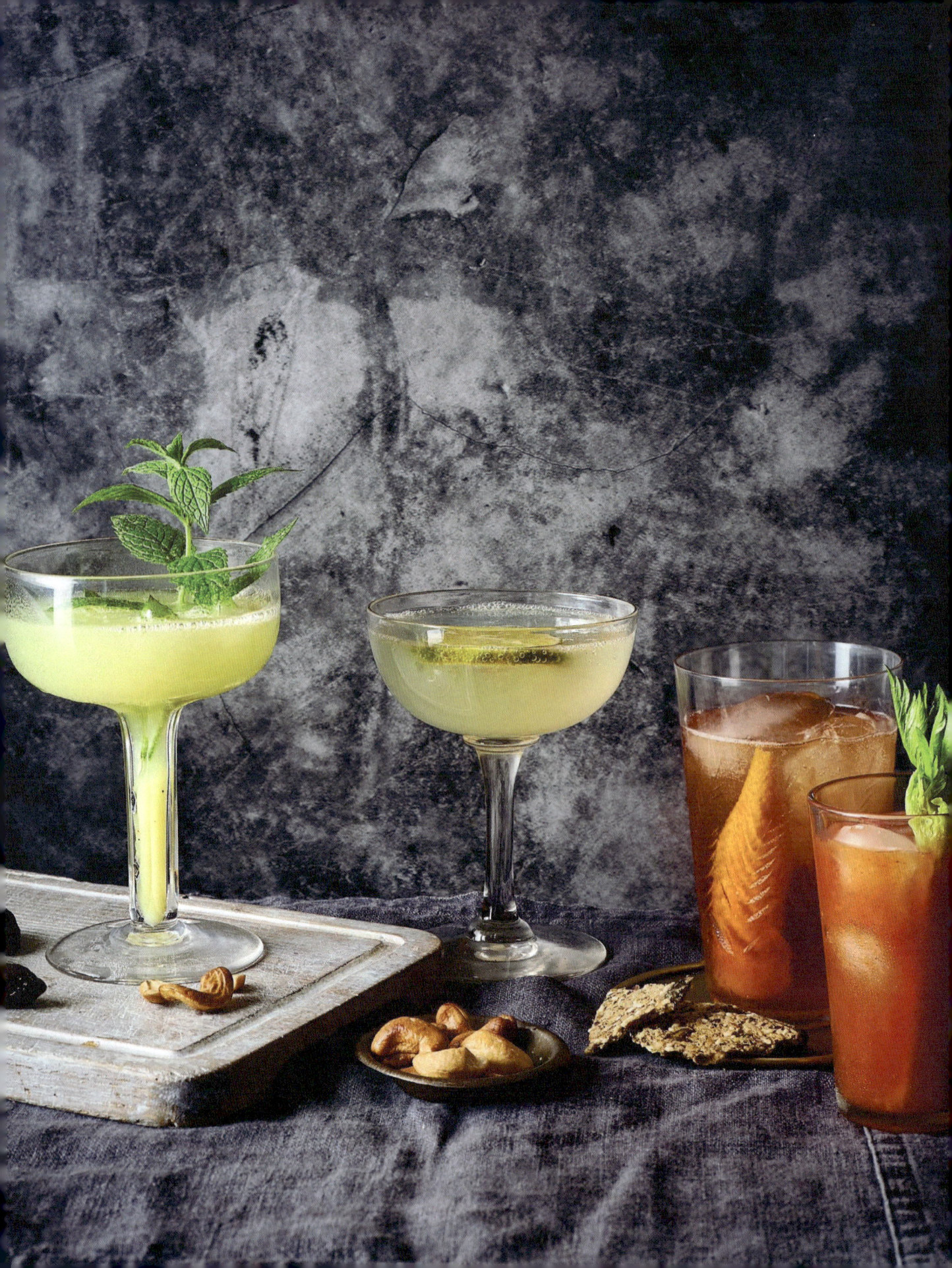

Ginger Sparkler

I used to love the small bottles of ginger shots you can buy but when I looked at the ingredients, I realized they are based on apple juice which is naturally sugary and not good for a low-carb diet. After experimenting, I realized how easy it was to make your own sugar-free ginger juice. Now there is always a bottle in our fridge; we love it on no-booze nights as it still has a kick from the heat of the ginger rather than from any alcohol. Top it up with still or sparkling water or add a splash of white or dark rum to make a rum and ginger cocktail.

Makes enough for 6 long sparkling ginger drinks

100g (3½oz) fresh ginger, peeled
still or sparkling water
ice
sprig of mint

Whizz the ginger and 100ml (3½fl oz) water together in a blender and then strain the juice through a fine sieve into a jug. Discard the fibrous ginger left in the sieve. Pour the juice into a bottle or jar with a lid and store in the fridge for up to a week.

To make a Ginger Sparkler, mix 2 tablespoons of the ginger juice with still or sparkling water in a long glass and add ice and a sprig of mint.

Per serving of Ginger Sparkler: 2.1g net carbs, 0g fibre, 0.2g protein, 0.1g fat, 9kcal
Get ahead: The ginger juice keeps well in a jar in the fridge for up to a week. Stir through or shake before use.

Lime Soda

This is a simple and refreshing drink to have at any time of day and gives flavour and fizz even when you are avoiding alcohol. It's ideal to use up the leftover lime after you have made the [Coconut, Rum & Lime Trifle.](#)

Severs 1

2 tablespoons of lime juice with
100ml (3½fl oz) sparkling water

Mix the lime juice and the sparkling water together for a refreshing non-alcoholic drink.

Per serving: 2.4g net carbs, 0.1g fibre, 0.1g protein, 0g fat, 8kcal
Get ahead: Lime juice can be squeezed up to 3 days in advance and kept in the fridge or frozen until needed.

Glühwein

Mulled wine makes your house smell Christmassy and traditional on a cold winter's night. I suggest making this without any honey but to please a crowd add the minimum amount just to take the edge off any bitterness. It will still be a lot less sugar heavy than traditional mulled wine.

Serves 10

3 long strips of orange zest with no white pith, plus juice of 1 orange
1 apple, cored and cut into 2cm (¾in) cubes
a thumb-sized piece of fresh ginger, peeled and sliced
1 stick cinnamon
1 star anise
4 cloves
125ml (4fl oz) brandy
1 bottle of fruity red wine, such as Merlot
2 teaspoons mild honey or erythritol, to taste

Put all the ingredients into a large saucepan with 400ml (14fl oz) water over a low heat and warm for 15 minutes or until piping hot. Don't let it boil or you will burn away the alcohol. Transfer into heatproof glasses with a ladle, making sure everyone has a little fruit. You can pick out the cloves or warn your guests accordingly.

Per serving with honey: 5.2g net carbs, 0.4g fibre, 0.1g protein, 0g fat, 106cal
Per serving without honey: 4g net carbs, 0.4g fibre, 0.1g protein, 0g fat, 102kcal
Get ahead: The Glühwein can be prepared in the morning and left to steep in the fridge until you are ready to warm it through in the evening.

Whisky Oddball

This is a hybrid cocktail somewhere between a Whisky Highball and an Old Fashioned, invented by our son Giorgio for Giancarlo. Use a bourbon of your choice or change it to rum if you prefer. You will be pleased to know that whisky and other pure spirits don't contain carbs.

Serves 1

ice
½ teaspoon black treacle or honey or 2 teaspoons erythritol
60ml (4 tablespoons) bourbon
a good few dashes of Angostura bitters
Lemon wedge to serve
soda, to top

Use a teaspoon to mix the sweetener with the bourbon and Angostura bitters in a tumbler. Add the ice and drop in the wedge. Top up with the soda water.

Per serving: 1.9g net carbs, 0g fibre, 0.1g protein, 0g fat, 147kcal

Smoky Mary

This is an excellent way to use the Chilli Vodka if you made it for the Savoy Pasta with [Hot-smoked Salmon, Cream & Chilli Vodka.](#) This is our son Giorgio's recipe for this classic cocktail usually drunk in the morning. Apart from the natural sugars in the tomatoes, a Bloody Mary is one of the few sugar-free cocktails available and worth remembering the next time you are at the bar! We often blend a tin of Italian plum tomatoes in place of the tomato juice.

Serves 2

100ml (3½fl oz) chilli or normal vodka
400ml (14fl oz) tomato juice or blended tinned tomatoes
2 teaspoons lemon juice
¼ teaspoons smoked paprika
few drops of Tabasco
few drops of Worcestershire sauce
Half a teaspoon of celery salt
freshly ground black pepper
Pinch of salt
ice
2 small celery sticks

Mix all the ingredients together in a jug and adjust the seasoning to taste. Fill two glasses with ice, pour over the cocktail and garnish with the celery.

Per serving: 6.6g net carbs, 0.8g fibre, 1.7g protein, 0.6g fat, 150kcal

Get ahead: Mix the ingredients together and store in a jug in the fridge for up to a day. Pour over ice and add the celery just before serving.

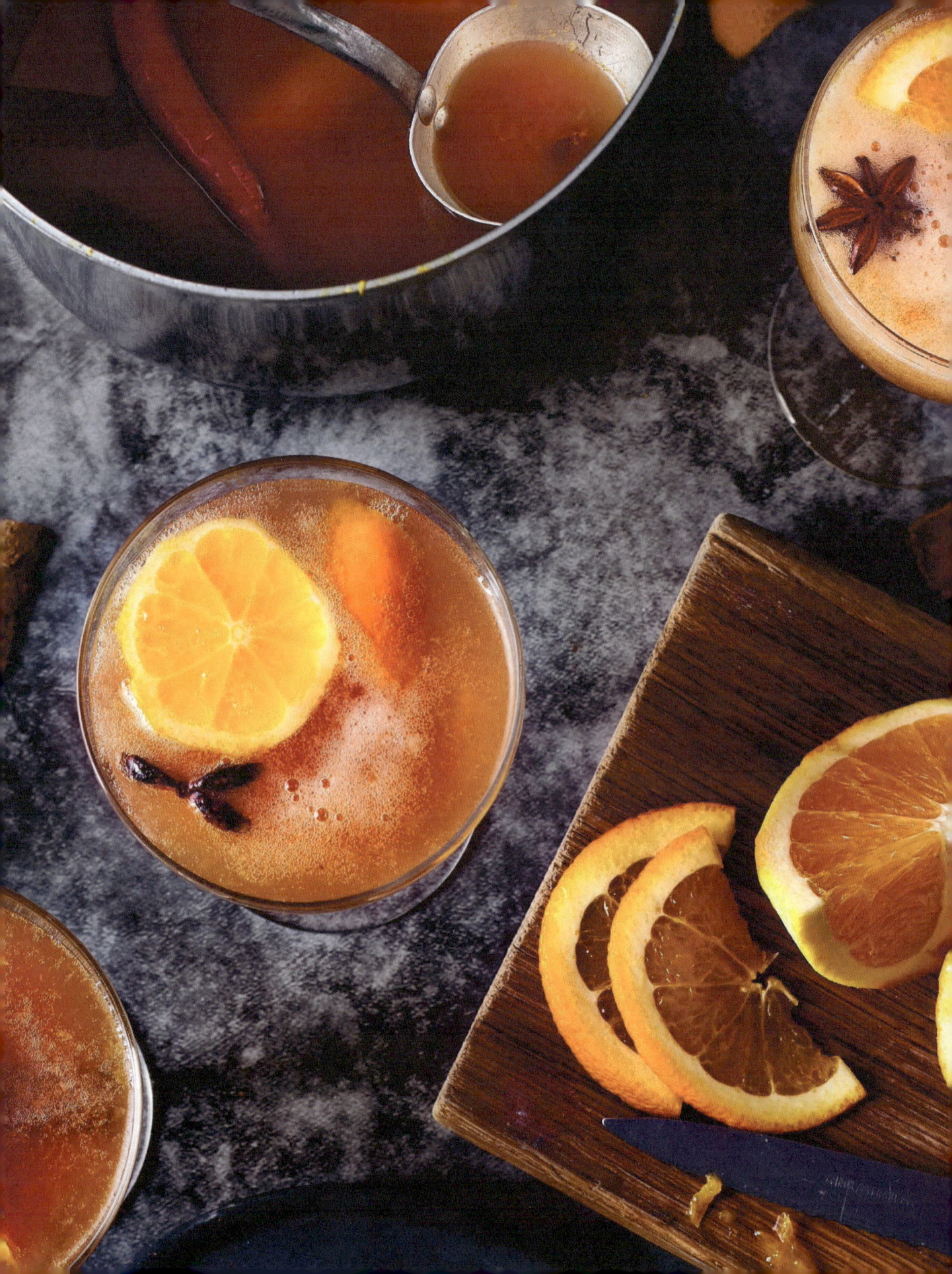

The Wonky Madonna

In a cocktail bar in Rome, I spotted a painting of a Madonna hanging askew on a dimly lit wall. She had obviously fallen at some point and had a plaster over her head to keep the canvas intact. Inspired by the painting's warm colours and durability, I created this innocent-tasting cocktail which has a hidden kick of chilli and alcohol. This recipe was originally written for our book Rome: Centuries in a Roman Kitchen but I have altered it to make a low-carb version. To make a non-alcoholic version, top up the spiced juice with soda water instead of the sparkling wine. A blood orange will give a richer colour if you can find them.

Makes 6 cocktails

1 bottle of dry sparkling wine, such as cava or champagne
6 tablespoons brandy
strips of orange zest
star anise and small cinnamon sticks, to serve (optional)
For the spiced orange juice
1 large blood or normal orange
1 small dried red chilli or ½ hot red chilli
5cm (2 in) cinnamon stick
1 star anise
3 cardamom pods, lightly crushed

To make the spiced orange juice, use a potato peeler to peel 9 long strips of orange zest from top to bottom of the orange. Put 3 of these in a medium saucepan and reserve the rest for the drinks. Squeeze the juice from the orange and add to the saucepan with the chilli, cinnamon stick, star anise, cardamom and 150ml (5fl oz) water. Bring to the boil, cook for a couple of minutes and crush the spices gently with a wooden spoon. Remove from the heat and leave to cool to room temperature. Cover and chill in the fridge to room temperature to infuse the flavours.

Pour the juice through a sieve into a jug and chill. When you are ready to serve, put a couple of ice cubes in 6 champagne glasses and mix 3 tablespoons of the spiced orange juice with 1 tablespoon of brandy in each glass. Top each glass with 100ml (3½fl oz) sparkling wine. Decorate the glasses with orange zest, star anise and cinnamon sticks as you like.

Per serving: 4.7g net carbs, 0g fibre, 0.2g protein, 0g fat, 143kcal

Get ahead: It is a good idea to make the spiced juice the night before you need it to allow the flavours to infuse. Once strained, it will keep in the fridge for 3 days.

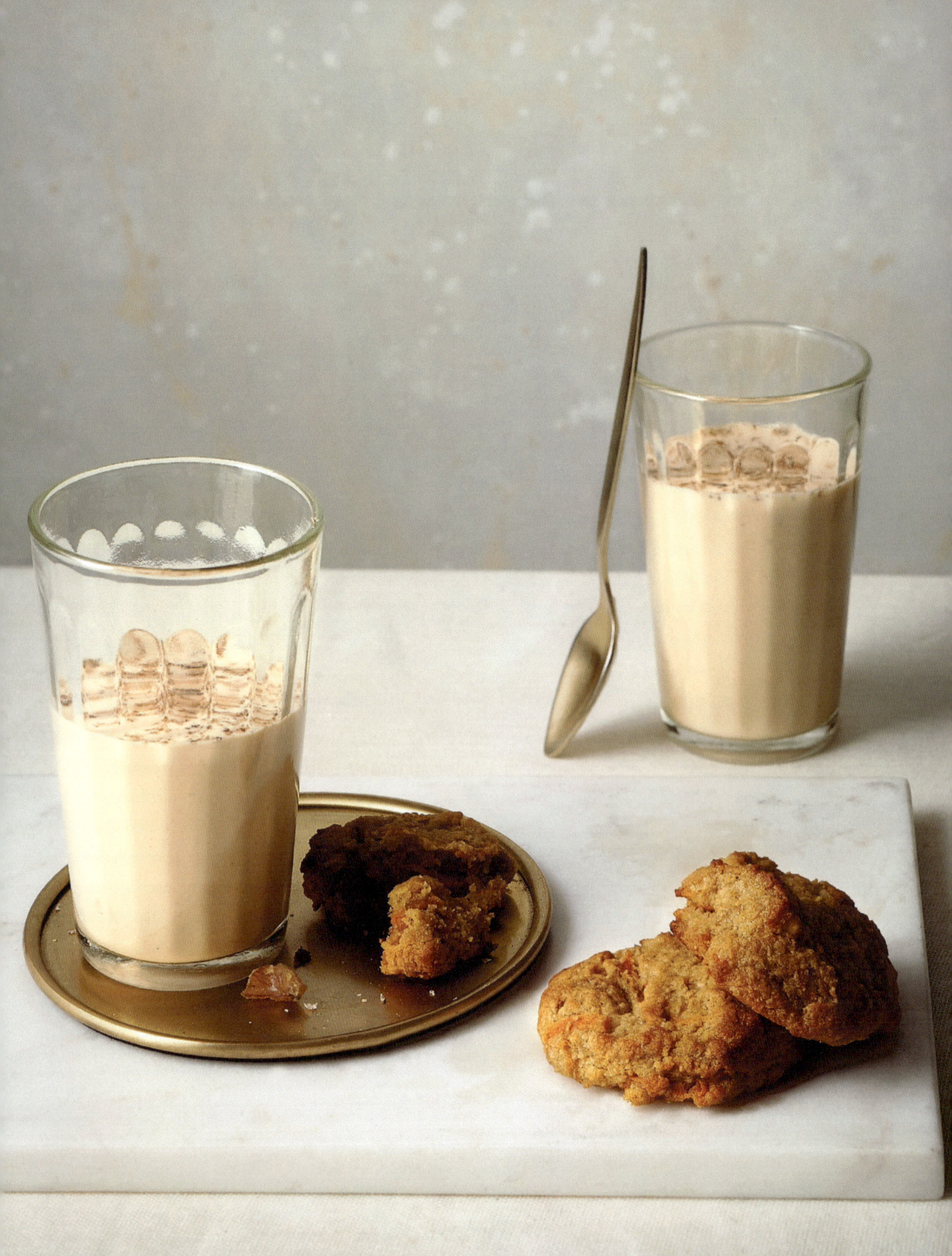

Eggnog

This creamy, innocent-looking drink packs a punch with rum and bourbon. Use minimal sweetener or leave it out completely if your sweet tooth has disappeared. To reduce the carbs further, use almond rather than cow's milk.

Serves 8/Makes 450ml (16fl oz)

200ml (7fl oz) cow's or almond milk
200ml (7fl oz double cream
2 egg yolks
1 teaspoon vanilla extract
40ml (3 tablespoons) rum
40ml (3 tablespoons) bourbon
2 teaspoons honey or 4 teaspoons erythritol
3cm (1¼in) cinnamon stick
grated nutmeg, to serve

Get a bowl of iced water ready. Whisk all the ingredients together in a saucepan until well blended. Put the saucepan over a gentle heat and keep whisking. Gradually increase the heat until the mixture starts to thicken and coats the back of a spoon. Remove from the heat and strain the mixture through a sieve into a bowl. Discard the cinnamon stick. Put this bowl over the bowl of iced water to chill it quickly.

Once cool, pour into a jug and cover. Keep in the fridge for up 3 days. Serve in small glasses with grated nutmeg over the top.

Per serving: 3.5g net carbs, 0g fibre, 2.1g protein, 10.8g fat, 137kcal

Get ahead: The Eggnog keeps in the fridge for up to 3 days. Cover the surface to stop it forming a skin and give it a good stir before serving.

Acknowledgements

Since this is my first e-book, I know I tried the patience of many and wanted to say a big thank you to all of you.

Giancarlo, Giorgio and Flavio – Thank you cooking with me, shopping, washing up and especially for trying yet another Christmas pudding and telling me which one you like!

Phoebe Pearson – You are a star. We love your photos and design. A huge thank you.

Vicky Orchard – Thank you so much for the advice and editing.

Stefano Borella – Thank you for not throwing the 39th mince pie or sausage roll at me.

Jim Davies – Thank you for making order out of my chaos.

Louise and Phil Ford – Thank you for being "on it" and sending guidance from afar.

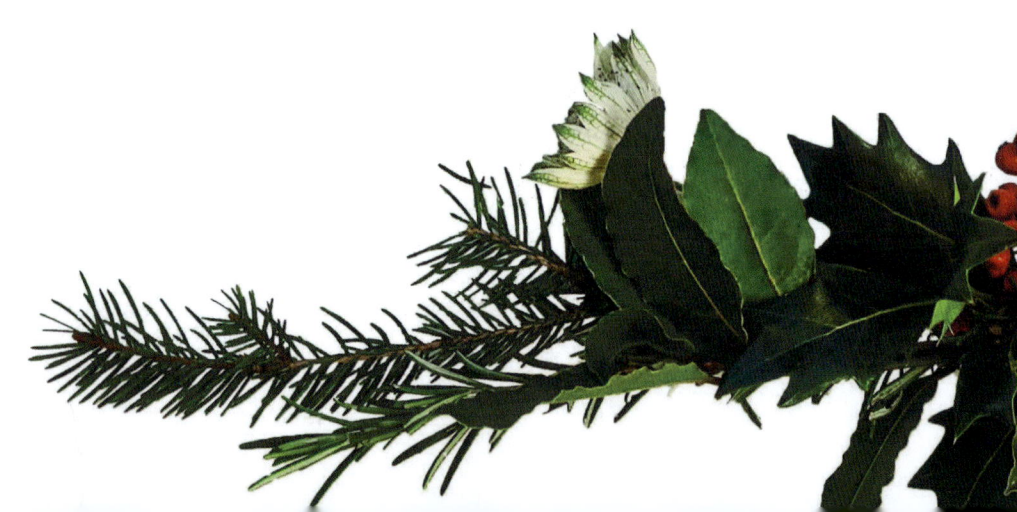